Advances in Kidney Transplantation

Advances in Kidney Transplantation

Guest Editors

Pedro Ruiz-Esteban

Domingo Hernández-Marrero

Verónica López-Jiménez

MDPI

Basel • Beijing • Wuhan • Barcelona • Belgrade • Novi Sad • Cluj • Manchester

Guest Editors
Pedro Ruiz-Esteban
Nephrology Department
Hospital Regional
Universitario de Málaga
Malaga
Spain

Domingo Hernández-Marrero
Nephrology Department
Hospital Universitario de Canarias
Tenerife
Spain

Verónica López-Jiménez
Nephrology Department
Hospital Regional
Universitario de Málaga
Malaga
Spain

Editorial Office
MDPI AG
Grosspeteranlage 5
4052 Basel, Switzerland

This is a reprint of the Special Issue, published open access by the journal *Journal of Clinical Medicine* (ISSN 2077-0383), freely accessible at: https://www.mdpi.com/journal/jcm/special_issues/0G263KQ0D0.

For citation purposes, cite each article independently as indicated on the article page online and as indicated below:

Lastname, A.A.; Lastname, B.B. Article Title. *Journal Name* **Year**, *Volume Number*, Page Range.

ISBN 978-3-7258-6966-4 (Hbk)
ISBN 978-3-7258-6967-1 (PDF)
https://doi.org/10.3390/books978-3-7258-6967-1

Contents

About the Editors

Pedro Ruiz-Esteban

Pedro Ruiz-Esteban holds a Bachelor's degree in Biology and a PhD from the University of Málaga. He is a researcher at the Nephrology Department, Hospital Universitario Regional de Málaga, Universidad de Málaga, Instituto de Investigación Biomédica de Málaga (IBIMA)-Plataforma BIONAND, RICORS2040-renal (RD24/0004/0026), specializing in nephrology and kidney transplantation. His primary areas include renal transplant outcomes, clinical trials in immunosuppression, and patient education in chronic kidney disease. He has authored 43 publications in kidney transplantation and participated in projects and trials funded by the Instituto de Salud Carlos III, Consejería de Salud de Andalucía, and scientific societies.

He has contributed to society through two popular science books: "Manual del paciente en diálisis y trasplante renal", emphasizing nutrition for chronic patients and leading to nutricionendialisis.com, and "Guía Integral de Nefrología: Comorbilidades, Complicaciones y Procesos Básicos", a guide for nephrology professionals and students. In researcher training, he collaborated on final degree projects in Medicine and Dermatology at the University of Málaga (2016–2018, 2024–2026) and was an Honorary Collaborator in Biochemistry (2016–2024), developing teaching materials.

He is part of research structures like RICORS2040 RD24/0004/0026, RD21/0005/0012, Emerging Group AE11-Nephrology at IBIMA (2023), REDiNREN RD16/0009/0006, and RD12/0021/0015. He has belonged to PAIDI CTS663: Nephrology and Kidney Transplantation (NTX) since 2011, previously CTS524 (2007–2011). He has supported projects like PAISIN on BK polyomavirus (2013–2015), T-regulatory lymphocytes in transplants (2011–2013), and calcineurin inhibitor studies (2009–2012). He holds three intellectual property registrations.

Domingo Hernández-Marrero

Domingo Hernández-Marrero holds a Medical Degree in Medicine and Surgery (1983) and a PhD from the University of La Laguna (1990). He currently serves as Head of the Nephrology Service at Hospital Universitario de Canarias and Full Professor in the Department of Internal Medicine, Dermatology, and Psychiatry at the University of La Laguna. Previously, he directed the Nephrology Clinical Management Unit at Hospital Regional Universitario de Málaga (2011–2023), held a Full Professorship in the Department of Medicine and Dermatology at the University of Málaga (2020–2023), coordinated the Kidney Transplantation Program of REDINREN (2014–2022), and was Scientific Vice-Director of IBIMA (2017–2022). He served as President of the Spanish Transplantation Society (SET) from 2018 to 2024 and currently leads the Canary Islands Transplantation Society.

As Principal Investigator, he leads key research groups including RICORS2040-Renal RD24/0004/0025, RICORS2040 RD21/0005/0012, REDINREN RD16/0009/0006 and RD12/0021/0015, PAIDI CTS-663, and the "Nephrology and Kidney Transplantation" group at IBIMA. He has earned 6 six-year research accreditation periods (1989–2024) and evaluates health research projects for the Instituto de Salud Carlos III and Andalucía's Health Department. Domingo has supervised 14 doctoral theses, led 14 competitive research projects, authored over 300 indexed publications, co-edited 5 books, and contributed to 43 book chapters.

He is a member of scientific committees for SET and the Spanish Society of Nephrology (SEN), served as Manager for Biomedicine-FIS projects at the State Research Agency (March-June 2020), and regularly reviews for top journals including *Nefrología*, *Transplantation*, *American Journal of*

Transplantation, *Journal of the American Society of Nephrology*, and *Kidney International*. His extensive leadership has advanced kidney transplantation research and clinical practice in Spain.

Verónica López-Jiménez

Verónica López-Jiménez holds a Medical Degree from the University of Granada (1999) and a PhD from the University of Málaga (2016). She works as Consultant Nephrologist at Hospital Regional Universitario de Málaga since 2005, specializing in kidney transplantation, and currently heads the Nephrology Department. She has participated in funded research projects and clinical trials by Instituto de Salud Carlos III and scientific societies, authoring over 80 JCR publications on transplantation. Her research focuses on immunosuppressive strategies, post-transplant complications (PI-0499, ICI14/00016), renal senescence (PI17/02043), and early inflammatory lesions (ICI21/00042), recently including SARS-CoV-2 effects in nephrology.

She has contributed to society by co-authoring clinical guidelines for transplant patients, especially during COVID-19, aiding evidence-based decisions. In training, she mentors medical students, MIR residents, and young nephrologists as Associate Professor and Coordinator of Medicine/Dermatology at University of Málaga, MIR Tutor, and Nephrology Specialty Coordinator at the hospital.

She belongs to research groups like RICORS RD24/0004/0026, RD21/0005/0012, REDINREN RD16/0009/0006, RD12/0021/0015, Emerging Group A-11 Nephrology at IBIMA, and PAIDI CTS663. As PI of AE-11 at IBIMA and RD24/0004/0026/RD21/0005/0012, she advances precision nephrology in transplantation for better outcomes.

Preface

The field of kidney transplantation faces ongoing challenges in optimizing patient outcomes while minimizing risks associated with immunosuppression and long-term graft survival. This Reprint addresses these critical issues through a curated collection of original research and reviews that explore innovative therapeutic strategies, biomarker development, and personalized clinical management. Our scope encompasses pharmacological advancements like finerenone and extended-release tacrolimus formulations, non-invasive monitoring tools such as Torque Teno virus load, and risk mitigation for complications including post-transplant diabetes, glomerular disease recurrence, and donor safety in complex anatomies.

The motivation for this scientific endeavor stems from the pressing need to translate emerging evidence into actionable clinical practices, particularly for high-risk populations like lung transplant recipients with end-stage renal disease and lactating patients on immunosuppression. As Guest Editors, we initiated this Special Issue to bridge gaps in current knowledge, fostering multidisciplinary dialogue among nephrologists, transplant surgeons, and pharmacologists worldwide. By compiling prospective cohort studies, randomized pilots, and narrative reviews, we aim to provide robust data supporting precision medicine approaches that enhance graft longevity and quality of life.

This Reprint is directed to clinicians, researchers, and policymakers in transplant nephrology seeking evidence-based insights to refine protocols and improve decision-making. It underscores the transformative potential of tailored therapies in reducing biopsy reliance and over-immunosuppression, ultimately advancing equitable access to superior post-transplant care.

Pedro Ruiz-Esteban, Domingo Hernández-Marrero, and Verónica López-Jiménez
Guest Editors

Journal of
Clinical Medicine

MDPI

Article

Efficacy of the Once-Daily Tacrolimus Formulation LCPT Compared to the Immediate-Release Formulation in Preventing Early Post-Transplant Diabetes in High-Risk Kidney Transplant Patients: A Randomized, Controlled, Open-Label Pilot Study (EUDRACT: 2017-000718-52)

Armando Torres [1,2,*], Concepción Rodríguez-Adanero [1], Constantino Fernández-Rivera [3], Domingo Marrero-Miranda [1], Eduardo de Bonis-Redondo [1], Aurelio P. Rodríguez-Hernández [1], Lourdes Pérez-Tamajón [1], Ana González-Rinne [1], Diego Álvarez-Sosa [1], Alejandra Álvarez-González [1], Nuria Sanchez-Dorta [1], Estefanía Pérez-Carreño [4], Laura Díaz-Martín [4], Sergio Luis-Lima [5], Ana E. Rodríguez-Rodríguez [2], Antonia María de Vera González [5], Cristina Romero-Delgado [6], María Calvo-Rodríguez [3], Rocío Seijo-Bestilleiro [3], Consuelo Rodríguez-Jiménez [7], Manuel Arturo Prieto López [1], Antonio Manuel Rivero-González [8], Domingo Hernández-Marrero [1,2] and Esteban Porrini [2]

1 Nephrology Service, Hospital Universitario de Canarias, 38320 La Laguna, Spain; c.rguez.adanero@gmail.com (C.R.-A.); dmarrero72@hotmail.com (D.M.-M.); ebonis@telefonica.net (E.d.B.-R.); aureliopas@hotmail.com (A.P.R.-H.); mpertam28@gmail.com (L.P.-T.); rinneanag@yahoo.es (A.G.-R.); diegoalvarezsosa@yahoo.es (D.Á.-S.); alejandramag73@gmail.com (A.Á.-G.); nuriasanchezdorta@gmail.com (N.S.-D.); manuloprieto1999@gmail.com (M.A.P.L.); domingohernandez@gmail.com (D.H.-M.)

2 Instituto de Tecnologías Biomédicas (ITB), Universidad de La Laguna, 38206 La Laguna, Spain; anarrguez@gmail.com (A.E.R.-R.); estebanporrini72@hotmail.com (E.P.)

3 Servicio de Nefrología, Complejo Hospitalario Universitario de A Coruña, 15006 La Coruña, Spain; constantino.fernandez.rivera@sergas.es (C.F.-R.); maria.calvo.rodriguez@sergas.es (M.C.-R.); rocio.seijo.bestilleiro@sergas.es (R.S.-B.)

4 Research Unit, Hospital Universitario de Canarias, 38320 La Laguna, Spain; estefaniaperezc@gmail.com (E.P.-C.); lauradiazmart@gmail.com (L.D.-M.)

5 Central Laboratory, Hospital Universitario de Canarias, 38320 La Laguna, Spain; luis.lima.sergio@gmail.com (S.L.-L.); adeverag@gmail.com (A.M.d.V.G.)

6 Pharmacy Service, Hospital Universitario de Canarias, 38320 La Laguna, Spain; cromdels@gobiernodecanarias.org

7 Pharmacology Service, Hospital Universitario de Canarias, 38320 La Laguna, Spain; conrodjim@gmail.com

8 Nephrology Service, Hospital Universitario Nuestra Señora de la Candelaria, 38010 Tenerife, Spain; arivero61@hotmail.com

* Correspondence: atorresram@gmail.com

Abstract: Background/Objectives: Post-transplant diabetes mellitus (PTDM) and prediabetes (PreDM) are common after renal transplantation and increase the risk of cardiovascular events and mortality. Compared to immediate-release tacrolimus (IR-Tac), the LCPT formulation, with delayed absorption, offers higher bioavailability and a smoother time–concentration curve, potentially reducing beta-cell stress. **Methods**: This randomized pilot trial compared de novo immunosuppression with IR-Tac (twice daily) and LCPT (once daily). At-risk recipients (age $\geq$ 60 years or 18–59 years with metabolic syndrome) were enrolled and followed for 3 months. The primary and secondary outcomes were the incidence of PTDM and PreDM, respectively. **Results**: 27 patients were randomized to IR-Tac and 25 to LCPT. The incidence of PTDM was comparable between groups [IR Tac: 18.5% (95% CI: 8.2–36.7%) vs. LCPT: 24% (95% CI: 11.5–43.4%); p = 0.7]. Although not statistically significant, the LCPT group exhibited a trend toward a reduction in PreDM incidence [IR-Tac: 40.7% (95% CI: 25–59%) vs. LCPT: 20% (95% CI: 9–39%); p = 0.1]. A sensitivity analysis showed similar results, with no significant differences in cumulative corticosteroid doses or baseline body mass index (BMI) between groups. The LCPT group showed a trend toward higher tacrolimus exposure at the end of the study [trough levels: IR-Tac group 8.3 (6.9–9.2) vs. LCPT group 9.4 (7.4–11.4) ng/mL; p = 0.05)], as well as fewer acute rejection episodes (none vs. three). Delayed graft function was more common in the IR-Tac group (37% vs. 8%; $p = 0.01$), and the eGFR was lower. Adverse events were comparable between groups. **Conclusions**: The potential biological activity of LCPT in preventing glucose metabolic alterations in at-risk patients warrants further investigation.

Keywords: kidney transplantation; post-transplant diabetes; post-transplant prediabetes; tacrolimus pharmacokinetics; early-release tacrolimus; LCPT tacrolimus

1. Introduction

Post-transplant diabetes mellitus (PTDM) is a serious condition affecting 10–30% of renal transplant recipients [1–3]. PTDM is linked to an increased risk of cardiovascular disease [4,5] and decreased patient survival [5]. Additionally, prediabetic states (PreDM: impaired glucose tolerance and/or impaired fasting glucose) are prevalent, with 40–50% of recipients developing PTDM or PreDM [2]. Recipients with PreDM also face a heightened risk of fatal or non-fatal cardiovascular events nearly equivalent to those with PTDM [4]. Mechanistically, a combination of insulin resistance and inefficient pancreatic beta-cell function predisposes individuals to PreDM and PTDM, with immunosuppression exacerbating pre-existing damage [3,6,7]. Tacrolimus, used in both animal models and human islets, exacerbates cellular damage caused by insulin resistance and obesity [8–10].

Different formulations of tacrolimus exhibit distinct pharmacokinetics. Immediate-release tacrolimus (IR-Tac), which is administered twice daily, is rapidly absorbed in the proximal small bowel, reaching peak blood concentrations 90 to 120 min post-administration. The once-daily extended-release tacrolimus (ER-Tac, Advagraf®, Astellas Pharma, Madrid, Spain) slows the diffusion rate of tacrolimus. Conversely, the once-daily LCPT tacrolimus, developed using MeltDose technology, results in a more distal distribution in the gut and delayed absorption. Compared to IR-Tac and ER-Tac, LCPT has a lower and delayed peak with comparable minimum concentrations and less peak-to-trough fluctuation [11–15]. LCPT also shows greater bioavailability, requiring 30% less dosing than IR-Tac and 36% less than ER-Tac [12]. However, a clear research gap exists regarding the clinical significance of this 'flatter' time–concentration curve of LCPT. We hypothesize that it may reduce beta-cell stress and, consequently, the incidence of PTDM and/or PreDM compared to a twice-daily formulation.

The aim of this pilot, randomized, open-label trial was to evaluate whether de novo immunosuppression with LCPT reduces the incidence of PTDM compared to IR-Tac. The incidence of PreDM was assessed as a secondary outcome. Patients at risk of PTDM [6] were included and followed for 3 months post-transplantation, a period associated with maximum beta-cell stress and peak incidence of PTDM [2]. To the best of our knowledge, this is the first randomized controlled study comparing these tacrolimus formulations.

2. Material and Methods

2.1. Study Design

This study was an investigator-driven, open-label, prospective, randomized phase IV clinical trial with a duration of 3 months. De novo renal transplant (RT) patients with low immunological risk and risk for PTDM were randomized 1:1 into two groups: IR-Tac (Prograf®, Astellas Pharma, Madrid, Spain) or LCPT tacrolimus (Envarsus®, Chiesi España, Barcelona, Spain). All participants received induction therapy with either basiliximab or rabbit thymoglobulin. Informed consent was obtained from all patients, and the study was approved by the Ethics and Clinical Research Committee of Hospital Universitario de Canarias. This study was Registered in the European Union Clinical Trials Register on 31 March 2017 (EUDRACT: 2017-000718-52).

2.2. Study Population

Two transplant centers participated in this study. The included patients had end-stage renal disease, received their first renal transplant (RT), and met the following "Metabolic Criteria": (a) recipient age $\geq$ 60 years or (b) recipient age between 18 and 59 years with metabolic syndrome (defined by the presence of at least three of the following criteria: BMI > 28 kg/m^2, treated hypertension, pre-transplant fasting glucose levels of 100–125 mg/dL, pre-transplant triglycerides levels $\geq$ 150 mg/dL, or HDL cholesterol levels < 40 mg/dL in men or <50 mg/dL in women). Exclusion criteria included pre-transplant diabetes (defined as baseline blood glucose level $\geq$ 126 mg/dL or the use of hypoglycemic medications), dual-organ transplantation, high immunological risk, infection with hepatitis B and/or C viruses, positive pregnancy test, or planned administration of non-standard immunosuppressive regimens (e.g., reduced tacrolimus exposure with mTOR inhibitors).

2.3. Randomization, Groups, and Interventions

After signing informed consent, patients were randomized 1:1 using a computerized algorithm generated by the Research Unit of Hospital Universitario de Canarias [16]. Due to the COVID-19 pandemic, the recruitment period was extended, beginning on 30 August 2017 and concluding on 5 April 2022.

- Group 1: IR-Tac: 0.1 mg/kg/day in 2 divided doses to maintain tacrolimus trough levels at between 8–12 ng/mL for the first month. A single dose of 0.05 mg/kg or 0.10 mg/kg (in expanded criteria or standard donor, respectively) was administered before surgery.
- Group 2: LCPT tacrolimus: 0.1 mg/kg/day in a single dose starting within the first 24 h after transplantation to maintain tacrolimus trough levels at between 8–12 ng/mL for the first month.

Doses of IR-Tac and LCPT were adjusted after the first month to maintain tacrolimus levels at between 6–10 ng/mL. Both groups also received additional immunosuppression with:

- Mycophenolate mofetil (MMF) 2 g/day or mycophenolic acid (EC-MFA) 1.44 g/day during the first month, then reduced to 1 g/day or 720 mg/day, respectively.
- Corticosteroids at reduced exposure as previously described, with slight modifications [16]: intravenous methylprednisolone 0.25 g intraoperatively and 60 mg on day 1; oral prednisone starting on day 3 with 20 mg/day, progressively reduced to 5 mg/day from day 42 until the end of the study.
- Induction was based on basiliximab, 20 mg intravenously on days 0 and 4. For grafts at high risk of delayed graft function (e.g., donation after cardiac death or prolonged cold ischemia time), a transient reduction of tacrolimus doses or delayed initiation (maximum of 5 days) plus induction with rabbit ATG was performed.

In cases of hyperglycemia in the early postoperative period, rapid insulin therapy was initiated when the fasting capillary blood glucose level was $\geq$160 mg/dL. Universal prophylaxis against Pneumocystis jirovecii was provided with cotrimoxazole (80 mg trimethoprym/400 mg sufamethoxazole/day, for 3 months), and cytomegalovirus (CMV) prophylaxis was given to at-risk patients with oral valganciclovir (450 mg/12 h if eGFR > 40 mL/mn/1.73 m^2, with the dosage adjusted appropriately for lower eGFR values). Biopsy-proven acute rejection was classified according to the Banff 2019 criteria [17] and treated with 3 boluses of 500 mg/day intravenous methylprednisolone. No corticosteroid-resistant or antibody-mediated rejection was observed during this study. Delayed graft function (DGF) was defined as the need for dialysis within the first week post-transplantation.

2.4. Assessment of Glucose Metabolism Alterations

Fasting blood glucose was measured at 1 week, 1 month, 2 months, and 3 months post-transplantation. A standard oral glucose tolerance test (OGTT) with 75 g glucose was performed at 3 months, except in patients who had already developed overt PTDM. Glucose and insulin levels were measured at baseline and after 30 and 120 min of glucose ingestion. Diabetes was defined according to ADA criteria [16] as fasting glucose > 125 mg/dL, the use of antidiabetic medication, or 2 h glucose $\geq$ 200 mg/dL. Impaired fasting glucose (IFG) was defined as fasting glucose $\geq$ 100 and <126 mg/dL, and impaired glucose tolerance (IGT) as 2 h glucose $\geq$ 140 and <200 mg/dL. IFG and IGT, isolated or combined, were considered prediabetic states (PreDM) [18]. The Insulin Sensitivity Index modified for renal transplant recipients (ISI-Tx) was calculated using the formula [6,19]: $0.208 - 0.0032 \times \text{BMI} - 0.0000645 \times \text{Ins } 120 - 0.00375 \times \text{Gluc } 120$, where Ins 120 and Gluc 120 are serum insulin (pmol/L) and plasma glucose (mmol/L) 120 min after the OGTT. The insulinogenic index (IGI) was calculated from insulin (μU/mL) and glucose (mmol/L) at 0 and 30 min and was used to estimate insulin secretory function: $(\text{Ins } 30 - \text{Ins } 0)/(\text{Gluc } 30 - \text{Gluc } 0)$ [6,20].

2.5. Analytical and Other Determinations

Plasma glucose, triglycerides, HDL, LDL cholesterol, and magnesium levels were determined using a clinical chemistry analyzer (Cobas-E 801, Roche Diagnostic, Barcelona, Spain®). Glycated hemoglobin (HbA1c) was measured by high-performance liquid chromatography (D-100; Biorad® Madrid, Spain). Insulin levels were measured using a chemiluminescence immunoassay system (Abbott Laboratories®, Madrid, Spain). The GFR was estimated by MDRD 4 (eGFR), and proteinuria was quantified either in 24 h urine or as the protein/creatinine ratio in the first voided morning sample by standard methods. At the end of the study, the GFR was measured by iohexol plasma clearance as previously described [21]. Whole-blood tacrolimus trough levels were determined by automated chemiluminescence assays with frequent determinations as per clinical practice (Architect Tacrolimus, Abbot, Madrid, Spain). Levels were also recorded at 1 week and at 1, 2, and 3 months.

At the end of the study, 24 h ambulatory blood pressure monitoring was performed on each group.

2.6. Efficacy Variables

The primary endpoint was the presence of PTDM based on ADA criteria. The incidence of PreDM (IGT and/or IFG) was assessed as a secondary outcome. Post-OGTT glucose levels were also compared between IR-Tac and LCPT groups. HbA1c was not included due to its lack of diagnostic sensitivity early after transplantation [3]. Major safety variables included biopsy-proven acute rejection rate, patient and graft survival, eGFR, and proteinuria. Treatment-emergent severe and non-severe side effects were recorded and reported to the Pharmacovigilance Unit of the Hospital Universitario de Canarias.

2.7. Statistical Analysis

Continuous variables are expressed as mean $\pm$ standard deviation or median plus interquartile range as appropriate; categorical variables are expressed as percentages. The Student's t-test or the Mann–Whitney U test, as appropriate, was used for comparisons of two independent samples. Categorical variables were compared using the chi-square test or Fisher's exact test. A p-value < 0.05 was considered statistically significant.

2.8. Sample Size

No comparison of IR-tacrolimus vs. LCPT with post-transplant glucose metabolic alterations as the primary endpoint has been conducted. Therefore, we planned a pilot study aimed at detecting a reduction of the composite of PTDM plus PreDM from the reported 52% three months after transplantation [2] to 20%. For a single-sided alpha of

0.05 and beta of 0.8, 27 patients per arm should be included. For this exploratory trial, we performed a per-protocol analysis.

2.9. Safety

Adverse events were monitored systematically and continuously. Serious adverse events were defined according to the International Conference on Harmonisation's Guideline for Clinical Safety Data Management. Treatment-emergent severe and non-severe side effects were recorded and reported to the Pharmacovigilance Unit of the Hospital Universitario de Canarias.

Major safety variables included the biopsy-proven acute rejection rate, patient and graft survival, eGFR, and proteinuria.

3. Results

3.1. Patient Disposition

Figure 1 illustrates the patients' disposition. A total of 62 patients were randomized, with 10 patients subsequently excluded (three from the IR-Tac group and seven from the LCPT group). The most common reason for exclusion was a violation of the immunosuppression protocol. Ultimately, 52 patients completed the study, with 27 in the IR-Tac group and 25 in the LCPT group.

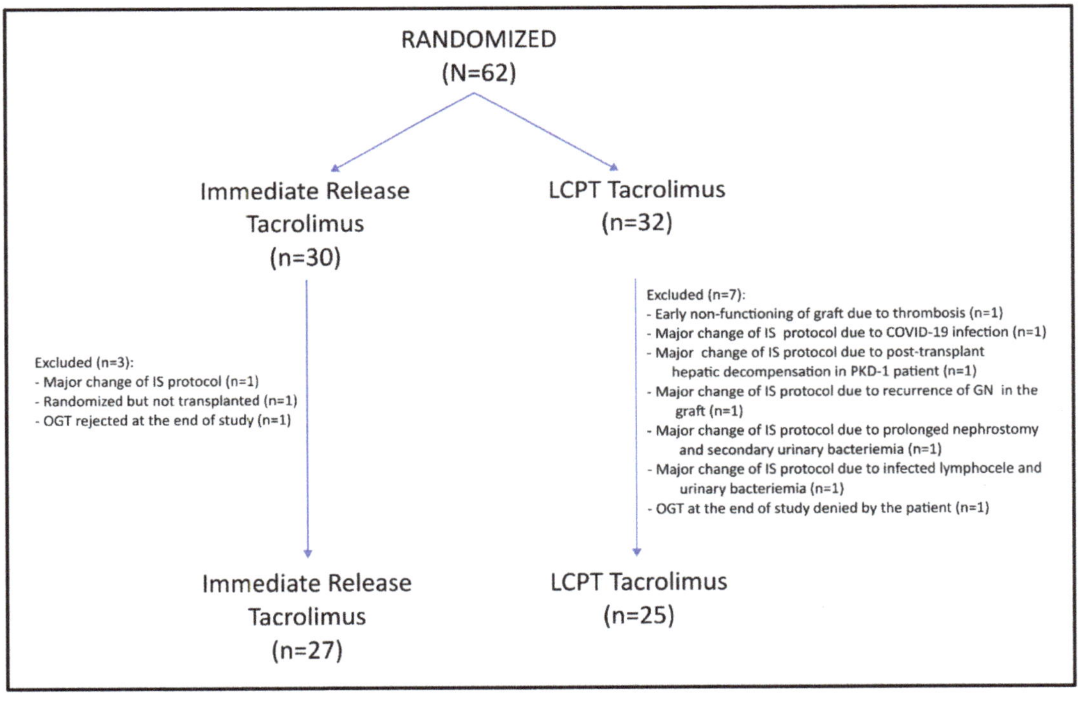

Figure 1. Patients' disposition. IS: Immunosuppression; OGT: Oral glucose tolerance test. PKD-1: Autosomal Dominant Polycystic Kidney Disease type I; GN: Glomerulonephritis.

3.2. Baseline Demographics of Recipients and Donors

Table 1 presents the baseline characteristics of recipients and donors in the two study groups. Variables associated with PTDM risk were balanced between the groups, except for BMI, which was higher in the IR-Tac group by chance. Delayed graft function was significantly more common in the IR-Tac group regardless of age, cold ischemia time, donor type (Table 1), or the use of r-ATG for induction (22.2% of patients in the IR-Tac group and 12% in the LCPT group (p = 0.5)).

Table 1. Baseline characteristics.

Variable	IR-TAC (n = 27)	LCPT (n = 25)	p-Value
Recipient Age (years)	64 (50.6–68.2)	63.52 (46.53–69.66)	0.7
Sex (% Males)	17/27 (63%)	19/25 (76%)	0.31
Race (% Caucasians)	26/27 (96.3%)	23/25 (92%)	0.58
BMI (Kg/m^2)	28.61 ± 4.43	25.53 ± 4.19	0.013
Family history of Diabetes	7/24 (29.2%)	9/23 (39.1%)	0.47
Polycystic kidney disease	5/27 (18.5%)	6/25 (24%)	0.63
Peritoneal dialysis	7/26 (26.9%)	12/25 (48%)	0.12
Time on dialysis (months)	21.9 (15.2–32)	23.4 (9.7–28.6)	0.8
Total Cholesterol (mg/dL)	152.92 ± 38.84 (n = 26)	158.59 ± 37.27 (n = 22)	0.61
HDL cholesterol (mg/dL)	43.62 ± 13.32 (n = 21)	44.10 ± 11.42 (n = 21)	0.90
LDL cholesterol (mg/dL)	75 (56–99) (n = 19)	67 (60–98.5) (n = 21)	0.9
Triglycerides (mg/dL)	143 (102–167.8) (n = 26)	145 (103.5–181.5) (n = 22)	0.7
Tobacco (former or current smoker)	8/26 (30.8%)	13/25 (52%)	0.30
Statin treatment	19/26 (73.1%)	17/25 (68%)	0.70
Fasting glucose (mg/dL)	90.3 (83–96)	91 (83.5–94.5)	0.8
HbA1c (%)	5.19 ± 0.41 (n = 18)	5.22 ± 0.29 (n = 17)	0.85
Donor age (years)	56.70 ± 10.67	55.24 ± 13.40	0.66
Donor Sex (% Males)	17/27 (63%)	20/25 (80%)	0.18
Cold Ischemia Time (hours)	11.42 (6.54–18.67)	10.12 (7.66–16.58)	0.99
Donation after cardiac death	8/27 (29.6%)	6/25 (24%)	0.65
Delayed graft function	10/27 (37%)	2/25 (8%)	0.02

IR-TAC: Immediate-release tacrolimus; LCPT: LCP Tacrolimus.

3.3. Post-Transplant Evolution and Other Outcomes at the End of the Study

As shown in Table 2, three cases of biopsy-proven acute rejection were observed in the IR-Tac group, while there were none in the LCPT group. Consequently, the cumulative corticosteroid dose at the end of the study was significantly higher in the IR-Tac group. CMV and BKV infections were comparable between the groups. Due to the lower incidence of delayed graft function (DGF) in the LCPT group (Table 1), the estimated glomerular filtration rate (eGFR) at one and two months was significantly higher in the LCPT group (Table 2). Although differences at 3 months did not reach statistical significance, the mean measured GFR was 6.2 mL/min higher in the LCPT arm (Table 2). Proteinuria levels were comparable between the groups. At the end of the study, there was a trend toward lower weight gain in the IR-Tac group (Table 2). Lipid levels, blood pressure, and magnesium levels were similar between the groups. None of the included patients lost their grafts, and all survived.

Table 2. Post-Renal-Transplantation evolution and other outcomes at the end of the study.

Variable	IR-TAC (n = 27)	LCTP (n = 25)	*p*-Value
BMI (Kg/m^2)	28.34 ± 4.64	26.02 ± 3.71	0.06
Weight increase (Kg)	−0.99 ± 4.1	0.92 ± 4.7	0.1
Total Cholesterol (mg/dL)	192.63 ± 38.52 (n = 24)	176.96 ± 40.17 (n = 23)	0.18
HDL cholesterol (mg/dL)	52.04 ± 15.24 (n = 23)	53.87 ± 16.92 (n = 23)	0.70
LDL cholesterol (mg/dL)	109.45 ± 32.16 (n = 20)	99.64 ± 33.63 (n = 22)	0.34
Triglycerides (mg/dL)	132 (101–170)	116 (100.50–143.50)	0.36
Statin therapy	9/26 (34.6%)	12/25 (48%)	0.33
Magnesium (1 week) Magnesium (1 month) Magnesium (2 months)	1.96 ± 0.3 1.55 ± 0.3 1.6 ± 0.16	1.9 ± 0.3 1.5 ± 0.15 1.6 ± 0.17	0.4 0.7 0.9
CNI-related acute nephrotoxicity (%)	0/27 (0%)	2/25 (8%)	0.2
Acute Rejection (%)	3/27 (11.1%)	0/25 (0%)	0.2
Cumulative corticosteroid dose (mg)	1321.25 (1189.38–1561.25)	1195 (1173.75–1270)	0.05
CMV Infection (%)	2/27 (9.4%)	2/25 (8%)	1
BKV Infection (%)	0%	1/25 (4%)	0.8
Awake SPB (ABPM) (mmHg)	129.60 ± 12.55 (n = 25)	129.84 ± 12.78 (n = 25)	0.95
Asleep SBP (ABPM) (mmHg)	124.68 ± 13.19 (n = 25)	129.48 ± 16.92 (n = 25)	0.27
Awake DBP (ABPM) (mmHg)	79.92 ± 8.11 (n = 25)	80.48 ± 8.61 (n = 25)	0.81
Asleep DBP (ABPM) (mmHg)	75.32 ± 8.46 (n = 25)	77.80 ± 8.75 (n = 25)	0.31
Creatinine (mg/dL) 1 month 2 months 3 months	 1.77 (1.48–2.48) 1.65 (1.43–1.95) 1.6 (1.36–1.86)	 1.52 (1.28–1.75) 1.46 (1.2–1.85) 1.42 (1.14–1.87)	 0.07 0.1 0.36
eGFR (mL/mn/1.73 m^2) 1 month 2 months 3 months	 39.23 ± 16.57 41.16 ± 14.36 44.68 ± 13.99	 49.16 ± 15.74 48.92 ± 13.95 51.28 ± 15.48	 0.03 0.05 0.11
Measured GFR 3 months (mL/mn)	49.2 ± 17.3 (n = 26)	55.4 ± 18.2 (n = 23)	0.2
Proteinuria 3 months (mg/gr creatinine)	154.2 (133.2–244.2)	152.8 (139.7–271.2)	0.90

IR-TAC: Immediate-release tacrolimus; LCPT: LCP Tacrolimus. CNI: calcineurin inhibitor. CMV: Cytomegalovirus. BKV: BK virus. ABPM: 24 h ambulatory blood pressure monitoring. SBP: systolic blood pressure; DBP: diastolic blood pressure. eGFR: estimated GFR (MDRD).

3.4. *Tacrolimus Exposure*

Tacrolimus trough levels were similar throughout the study in both groups, except at 3 months when they were higher in the LCPT group (Table 3). At this time point, a higher proportion of patients in the LCPT group exhibited tacrolimus levels above the target range (7.4% vs. 40%; $p = 0.005$). Two cases of biopsy-proven acute reversible tacrolimus-related nephrotoxicity were observed in the LCPT group, while none were observed in the IR-Tac group (Table 2).

Table 3. Tacrolimus trough levels during the study.

Whole-Blood Tacrolimus Levels (ng/mL)	IR-Tacrolimus (n = 27)	LCPT (n = 25)	p-Value
1 week	9.5 (7.1–12.9)	10.5 (9.4–14.5)	0.1
1 month	9.5 (7.5–11.2)	9.8 (7.6–11.7)	1
2 months	9.6 (7–12)	10.7 (8.3–13)	0.2
3 months	8.3 (6.9–9.2)	9.4 (7.4–11.4)	0.05

3.5. Primary and Secondary Efficacy Endpoints

Transient insulin therapy early after transplantation was comparable between groups: 19 out of 27 patients (70.4%) in the IR-Tac group and 13 out of 25 patients (59.4%) in the LCPT group (p = 0.26). Fasting glucose throughout the study was not significantly different between the groups (Table 4). Plasma glucose levels 30 min after the OGTT were significantly lower in the LCPT group (Table 4).

Table 4. Primary and secondary outcomes for each group.

Variables	IR-TAC (n = 27)	LCPT (n = 25)	p-Value
Fasting Glucose (mg/dL):			
Pre-Transplantation	90.3 (83–96)	91 (83.5–94.5)	0.77
1 week	102 (92–116)	99 (93–116)	0.88
1 month	90 (83–98)	92 (86–104)	0.69
2 months	95 (86–108)	92 (85.25–105)	0.68
3 months	92 (86–102)	88 (81–97.5)	0.24
Oral Glucose Tolerance Test (3 months)			
Baseline Fasting Glycemia (mg/dL)	92 (86–102)	88 (81–97.5)	0.24
Glycemia at 30 min (mg/dL)	157 (138–178.50) (n = 18)	139 (125–154.5) (n = 21)	0.02
Glycemia at 120 mn (mg/dL)	131 (111–167) (n = 27)	120 (97–181) (n = 23)	0.53
Baseline Insulin (mcU/mL)	7.9 (4.8–10.2) (n = 23)	7 (5.5–10) (n = 23)	0.84
Insulin at 30 min (mcU/mL)	25.35 (13.95–41.23) (n = 18)	22.9 (9–43.6) (n = 21)	0.67
Insulin at 120 min (mcU/mL)	32.35 (16.1–49) (n = 22)	27.90 (7.1–44.5) (n = 23)	0.32
Insulin Sensitivity Index (ISI)	7.4 (5.7–8.8) (n = 22)	8.5 (6.6–9.8) (n = 23)	0.2
Insulinogenic Index	43.7 (20.7–66.4) (n = 16)	38.4 (22.7–147.2) (n = 19)	0.7
DISTRIBUTION OF GLUCOSE METABOLIC ALTERATIONS AT THE END OF STUDY			
Normal Tolerance	11/27 (40.7%) (95%CI: 24.5–59%)	14/25 (56%) (95%CI: 37.1–73.3%)	0.4
Isolated impaired fasting glucose (IFG)	3/27 (11.1%) (95%CI: 3.85–28.1%)	1/25 (4%) (95%CI: 0.7–19.5%)	0.6
Impaired Glucose Tolerance (IGT)	8/27 (29.6%) (95%CI: 15.9–48.5%)	4/25 (16%) (95%CI: 6.4–34.7%)	0.3
Post-transplant diabetes	5/27 (18.5%) (95%CI: 8.2–36.7%)	6/25 (24%) (95%CI: 11.5–43.4%)	0.7
Prediabetes (IFG + IGT)	11/27 (40.7%) (95%CI: 25–59%)	5/25 (20%) (95%CI: 9–39%)	0.1

PTDM incidence was comparable between the groups (Table 4). However, normal glucose tolerance was numerically more common in the LCPT group (56% vs. 40.7%), occurring at the expense of a 50% reduction in prediabetic states (IGT and/or IFG), which did not reach statistical significance (p = 0.1) (Table 4; Figure 2A).

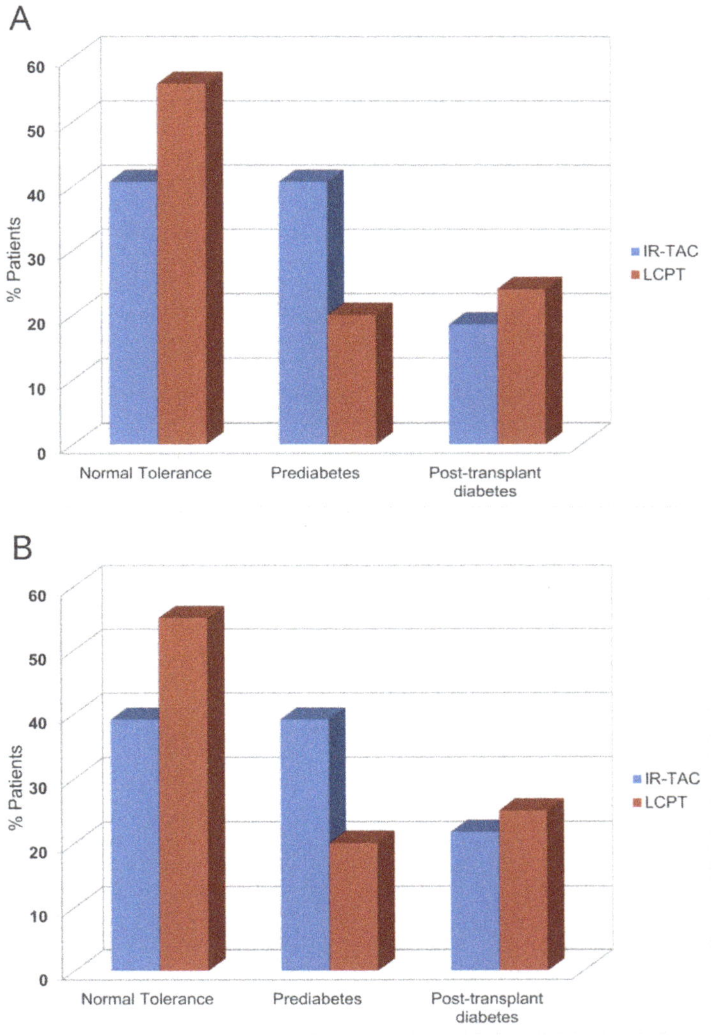

Figure 2. Distribution of glucose metabolism abnormalities at the end of the study in each group. Prediabetes: Impaired Fasting Glucose and Impaired Glucose Tolerance, isolated or combined. (**A**): All patients; (**B**): Excluding patients with acute rejection or a baseline BMI < 22 Kg/m^2. IR-Tac: Immediate-release tacrolimus; LCPT: LCP Tacrolimus.

3.6. Sensitivity Analysis

Since all biopsy-proven acute rejections occurred in the IR-Tac group, the cumulative corticosteroid dose was higher in this group (Table 2). Additionally, by chance, baseline BMI was significantly higher in the IR-Tac group (Table 1). These differences became non-significant when excluding patients with acute rejection or the lowest values of baseline BMI ($\leq$10th percentile: $\leq$22 kg/m^2), who likely exhibit lower insulin resistance and chances of developing tacrolimus-induced PTDM or PreDM [6,8] (Supplementary Table S1).

Notably, the differences in primary and secondary outcomes between the groups remained unchanged (Supplementary Table S1; Figure 2B).

3.7. Adverse Events

The total number of severe and non-severe adverse events was comparable between the groups (Supplementary Table S2). In the analysis stratified by gender, urinary tract infections and overall infectious episodes were significantly lower in women in the LCPT group.

4. Discussion

Immediate-release tacrolimus (IR-Tac) is rapidly absorbed in the proximal small bowel, achieving peak blood concentrations 90 to 120 min after administration twice daily. This 3-month randomized pilot study investigated whether the "flatter" concentration–time curve of once-daily tacrolimus (LCPT) could mitigate beta-cell stress and glucose metabolism disturbances following renal transplantation, especially among recipients at risk for post-transplant prediabetes (PreDM) or diabetes (PTDM) [1,6,7], evaluated at the peak incidence of glucose metabolism disorders (3 months post-transplant) [2].

To our knowledge, no study has examined the clinical significance of different tacrolimus pharmacokinetics on glucose metabolism after transplantation. Thus, this pilot and exploratory study was designed with a sample size to detect a 60% reduction in combined PTDM or PreDM incidence [2]. This aimed to provide initial insight into whether LCPT might exhibit a lower incidence of glucose metabolism disorders, guiding future trials with adequate statistical power.

Plasma glucose levels following an OGTT at the study's conclusion were numerically lower in the LCPT group, achieving statistical significance at 30 min (Table 4). Consequently, the incidence of glucose metabolism disorders at 3 months post-transplantation was reduced by 15% with LCPT, primarily due to a 50% decrease in PreDM, while no advantage was observed in PTDM incidence (Table 4; Figure 2A). This outcome may be attributed to the heightened susceptibility of patients with severely impaired beta-cell function pre-transplant to developing PTDM after exposure to tacrolimus [6], irrespective of formulation. In contrast, LCPT's smoother pharmacokinetic profile is expected to mitigate PreDM incidence in cases of less severe beta-cell damage. The trend toward a reduction in PreDM observed in this study is noteworthy, as PreDM substantially increases long-term mortality [5], poses a cardiovascular risk almost equivalent to that of PTDM [4], and is a risk factor for the subsequent development of PTDM [2]. However, this finding has to be confirmed in future adequately powered studies. Lastly, these differences in glucose metabolism favoring LCPT were noted alongside a trend towards higher tacrolimus exposure (Table 3) and improved efficacy (lower incidence of acute rejection; Table 2).

Baseline risk factors such as a family history of diabetes, age, race, magnesium levels, or statin use [1,3,6] were balanced between groups. However, chance imbalances in pre-transplant BMI and acute rejection episodes (all occurring in the IR-Tac group) were notable confounders. Sensitivity analysis excluding patients with acute rejection or a BMI < 22 Kg/m^2 indicated persistent between-group differences in glucose metabolism, with comparable BMI and cumulative steroid doses (Supplementary Table S1; Figure 2B), suggesting LCPT's potential benefits independent of these factors.

The incidence of DGF was significantly lower with LCPT (Table 2). This was not attributable to differences in donor age, cold ischemia time, donor type, or induction therapy with rabbit ATG. This difference may partly stem from the timing of tacrolimus initiation. IR-Tac was started just before RT and may have contributed to ischemia-reperfusion injury, whereas LCPT was administered within 24 h post-transplantation. Additionally, the better preservation of residual renal function in PD patients, who were more prevalent in the LCPT group (Table 1), may have contributed to the reduction in DGF. As a result of the lower incidence of DGF, better renal function was observed in the LCPT group during the first two months, although this significance diminished by three months (Table 2).

Total severe and non-severe adverse events were comparable between groups (Supplementary Table S2). In a gender-stratified analysis, rates of urinary tract infections were significantly lower among women in the LCPT group. We acknowledge that without controlling for confounding variables such as the duration of bladder catheterization or ureteral stent placement, we cannot draw definitive conclusions.

This study acknowledges several limitations. Due to its exploratory nature, this study included a limited number of patients, was conducted over a relatively short period, and lacked the statistical power necessary to support recommending LCPT for the management of glucose metabolism disorders in clinical practice (beta 0.28 for an alpha of 0.05). The small sample size was likely a significant factor contributing to the unbalanced randomization of baseline BMI. The cumulative corticosteroid dose was also unevenly distributed between the groups, as all three acute rejection episodes observed in this study occurred within the IR-Tac group. Although these imbalances were addressed through a sensitivity analysis, the possibility of bias cannot be ruled out. Nonetheless, the study results indicate a promising direction, warranting further investigation into LCPT's potential biological activity. This trial lacked a formal pharmacokinetic study to support differences in Cmax and Tmax between the two formulations. A protocol biopsy at the end of the study was not planned but could have provided morphological insights into observed graft function differences. The majority of the patients were Caucasian, so the results cannot be extrapolated to other races. The study duration was extended due to overlap with the COVID-19 pandemic, reducing transplant activity. Lastly, findings may not apply to the once-daily extended-release formulation Advagraf®, which differs in its pharmacokinetic profile from LCPT [12,13].

In conclusion, this exploratory trial did not succeed in demonstrating a reduction in diabetes following renal transplantation in at-risk patients treated with LCPT. Nevertheless, it does suggest that LCPT may lower the incidence of prediabetes compared to IR-Tac. The potential biological effects of LCPT in preventing glucose metabolism disorders warrant further investigation.

Supplementary Materials: The following supporting information can be downloaded at: https://www.mdpi.com/article/10.3390/jcm13247802/s1, Table S1: Sensitivity analysis; Table S2: Adverse events.

Author Contributions: Conceptualization: A.T., E.P. and C.F.-R.; Methodology: A.T., E.P., C.R.-A., D.H.-M., S.L.-L., A.E.R.-R. and A.M.d.V.G.; Software: A.T., E.P. and D.H.-M.; Validation: A.T., E.P., C.F.-R. and C.R.-J.; Formal Analysis: A.T., D.M.-M., D.H.-M. and M.A.P.L.; Investigation: C.R.-A., D.M.-M., E.d.B.-R., A.P.R.-H., L.P.-T., A.G.-R., D.Á.-S., A.Á.-G., N.S.-D., M.C.-R., R.S.-B. and A.M.R.-G.; Data Curation: A.T., C.R.-A., D.M.-M., E.P.-C., L.D.-M. and M.A.P.L.; Writing original: A.T., D.H.-M. and D.M.-M.; Supervision: A.T., C.F.-R., E.P.-C., L.D.-M., C.R.-J., M.C.-R. and R.S.-B.; Project administration: A.T., E.P., E.P.-C., L.D.-M., C.R.-D., M.C.-R. and R.S.-B.; Funding acquisition: A.T., E.P. and D.H.-M. All authors have read and agreed to the published version of the manuscript.

Funding: This study was supported by research funding from the Nephrology Department at Hospital Universitario de Canarias (Fundación Bioavance, FBIO 2024.001).

Institutional Review Board Statement: The study was conducted in accordance with the Declaration of Helsinki and approved by the Ethics Committee of the Hospital Universitario de Canarias (CEIm): Spanish Registry protocol code: 2017-000718-52; local code: DMPT17; date of approval: 9 May 2017).

Informed Consent Statement: Informed consent was obtained from all subjects involved in the study.

Data Availability Statement: The data presented in this study are available on request from the corresponding author.

Acknowledgments: We are grateful to the kidney transplant teams of the hospitals involved in the study. This work has been carried out with the support without financial assistance of the Spanish Clinical Research and Clinical Trials Platform, SCReN (Spanish Clinical Research Network), funded by the Instituto de Salud Carlos III (ISCIII-General Subdirectorate for Evaluation and Promotion of Research, through project PT20/00051, integrated into the 2017–2020 National R&D&I Plan, and co-financed by the European Regional Development Fund (ERDF). Support without financial assistance was also obtained from RICORS RD24/0004/0025 and ICI 121/00042 from ISCIII, and EU Project DOKI-Diabetes, Obesity and the Kidney, PN:101079207 of the call: HORIZON-WIDERA-2021-ACCESS-03, Twinning.

Conflicts of Interest: The authors declare that they have no known competing financial interests or personal relationships that could have appeared to influence the work reported in this paper. AT has received honoraria from Alnylam and Chiesi for delivering scientific or educational presentations.

References

1. Jenssen, T.; Hartmann, A. Post-transplant diabetes mellitus in patients with solid organ transplants. *Nat. Rev. Endocrinol.* **2019**, *15*, 172–188. [CrossRef] [PubMed]
2. Porrini, E.L.; Díaz, J.M.; Moreso, F.; Delgado Mallen, P.I.; Torres, I.S.; Ibernon, M.; Bayés-Genís, B.; Benitez-Ruiz, R.; Lampreabe, I.; Lauzurrica, R.; et al. Clinical evolution of post-transplant diabetes mellitus. *Nephrol. Dial. Transplant.* **2016**, *31*, 495–505. [CrossRef] [PubMed]
3. Sharif, A.; Chakkera, H.; de Vries, A.P.J.; Eller, K.; Guthoff, M.; Haller, M.C.; Hornum, M.; Nordheim, E.; Kautzky-Willer, A.; Krebs, M.; et al. International consensus on post-transplantation diabetes mellitus. *Nephrol. Dial. Transplant.* **2024**, *39*, 531–549. [CrossRef] [PubMed] [PubMed Central]
4. Porrini, E.; Díaz, J.M.; Moreso, F.; Lauzurrica, R.; Ibernon, M.; Torres, I.S.; Ruiz, R.B.; Rodríguez Rodríguez, A.E.; Mallén, P.D.; Bayés-Genís, B.; et al. Prediabetes is a risk factor for cardiovascular disease following renal transplantation. *Kidney Int.* **2019**, *96*, 1374–1380. [CrossRef] [PubMed]
5. Valderhaug, T.G.; Hjelmesæth, J.; Hartmann, A.; Røislien, J.; Bergrem, H.A.; Leivestad, T.; Line, P.D.; Jenssen, T. The association of early post-transplant glucose levels with long-term mortality. *Diabetologia* **2011**, *54*, 1341–1349. [CrossRef] [PubMed]
6. Fariña-Hernández, A.; Marrero-Miranda, D.; Perez-Carreño, E.; De Vera-Gonzalez, A.; González, A.; Acosta-Sorensen, C.; Rodríguez-Rodríguez, A.E.; Collantes, T.; García, M.D.P.; Rodríguez-Muñoz, A.I.; et al. Pretransplant evaluation and the risk of glucose metabolic alterations after renal transplantation: A prospective study. *Nephrol. Dial. Transplant.* **2023**, *38*, 778–786. [CrossRef]
7. Rodríguez-Rodríguez, A.E.; Porrini, E.; Hornum, M.; Donate-Correa, J.; Morales-Febles, R.; Khemlani Ramchand, S.; Molina Lima, M.X.; Torres, A. Post-Transplant Diabetes Mellitus and Prediabetes in Renal Transplant Recipients: An Update. *Nephron* **2021**, *145*, 317–329. [CrossRef] [PubMed]
8. Rodriguez-Rodriguez, A.E.; Triñanes, J.; Velazquez-Garcia, S.; Porrini, E.; Vega Prieto, M.J.; Diez Fuentes, M.L.; Arevalo, M.; Salido Ruiz, E.; Torres, A. The higher diabetogenic risk of tacrolimus depends on pre-existing insulin resistance. A study in obese and lean Zucker rats. *Am. J. Transplant.* **2013**, *13*, 1665–1675. [CrossRef] [PubMed]
9. Triñanes, J.; Rodriguez-Rodriguez, A.E.; Brito-Casillas, Y.; Wagner, A.; De Vries, A.P.J.; Cuesto, G.; Acebes, A.; Salido, E.; Torres, A.; Porrini, E. Deciphering Tacrolimus- Induced Toxicity in Pancreatic beta Cells. *Am. J. Transplant.* **2017**, *17*, 2829–2840. [CrossRef] [PubMed]
10. Teixidó-Trujillo, S.; Porrini, E.; Menéndez-Quintanal, L.M.; Torres-Ramírez, A.; Fumero, C.; Rodríguez-Rodríguez, A.E. Induction of diabetes by Tacrolimus in a phenotypic model of obesity and metabolic syndrome. *Front. Endocrinol.* **2024**, *15*, 1388361. [CrossRef] [PubMed] [PubMed Central]
11. Gaber, A.O.; Alloway, R.R.; Bodziak, K.; Kaplan, B.; Bunnapradist, S. Conversion from twice-daily tacrolimus capsules to once-daily extended-release tacrolimus (LCPT): A phase 2 trial of stable renal transplant recipients. *Transplantation* **2013**, *96*, 191–197. [CrossRef] [PubMed] [PubMed Central]
12. Tremblay, S.; Nigro, V.; Weinberg, J.; Woodle, E.S.; Alloway, R.R. A Steady-State Head to-Head Pharmacokinetic Comparison of All FK-506 (Tacrolimus) Formulations (ASTCOFF): An Open-Label, Prospective, Randomized, Two-Arm, Three-Period Crossover Study. *Am. J. Transplant.* **2017**, *17*, 432–442. [CrossRef] [PubMed]
13. Oberbauer, R.; Bestard, O.; Furian, L.; Maggiore, U.; Pascual, J.; Rostaing, L.; Budde, K. Optimization of tacrolimus in kidney transplantation: New pharmacokinetic perspectives. *Transplant. Rev.* **2020**, *34*, 100531. [CrossRef] [PubMed]
14. Kamar, N.; Cassuto, E.; Piotti, G.; Govoni, M.; Ciurlia, G.; Geraci, S.; Poli, G.; Nicolini, G.; Mariat, C.; Essig, M.; et al. Pharmacokinetics of Prolonged-Release Once-Daily Formulations of Tacrolimus in de Novo Kidney Transplant Recipients: A Randomized, Parallel-Group, Open-Label, Multicenter Study. *Adv. Ther.* **2019**, *36*, 462–477. [CrossRef]
15. Trofe-Clark, J.; Brennan, D.C.; West-Thielke, P.; Milone, M.C.; Lim, M.A.; Neubauer, R.; Nigro, V.; Bloom, R.D. Results of ASERTAA, a Randomized Prospective Crossover Pharmacogenetic Study of Immediate-Release Versus Extended-Release Tacrolimus in African American Kidney Transplant Recipients. *Am. J. Kidney Dis.* **2018**, *71*, 315–326. [CrossRef] [PubMed]

16. Torres, A.; Hernández, D.; Moreso, F.; Serón, D.; Burgos, M.D.; Pallardó, L.M.; Kanter, J.; Díaz Corte, C.; Rodríguez, M.; Diaz, J.M.; et al. Randomized Controlled Trial Assessing the Impact of Tacrolimus Versus Cyclosporine on the Incidence of Posttransplant Diabetes Mellitus. *Kidney Int. Rep.* **2018**, *3*, 1304–1315. [CrossRef] [PubMed]
17. Loupy, A.; Haas, M.; Roufosse, C.; Naesens, M.; Adam, B.; Afrouzian, M.; Akalin, E.; Alachkar, N.; Bagnasco, S.; Becker, J.U.; et al. The Banff 2019 Kidney Meeting Report (I): Updates on and clarification of criteria for T cell- and antibody-mediated rejection. *Am. J. Transplant.* **2020**, *20*, 2318–2331. [CrossRef] [PubMed] [PubMed Central]
18. American Diabetes Association. 2. Classification and Diagnosis of Diabetes: Standards of Medical Care in Diabetes-2018. *Diabetes Care* **2018**, *41* (Suppl. S1), S13–S27. [CrossRef]
19. Hjelmesæth, J.; Midtvedt, K.; Jenssen, T.; Hartmann, A. Insulin resistance after renal transplantation: Impact of immunosuppressive and antihypertensive therapy. *Diabetes Care* **2001**, *24*, 2121–2126. [CrossRef]
20. Tura, A.; Kautzky-Willer, A.; Pacini, G. Insulinogenic indices from insulin and C-peptide: Comparison of beta-cell function from OGTT and IVGTT. *Diabetes Res. Clin. Pract.* **2006**, *72*, 298–301. [CrossRef] [PubMed]
21. Luis-Lima, S.; Gaspari, F.; Negrín-Mena, N.; Carrara, F.; Díaz-Martín, L.; Jiménez-Sosa, A.; González-Rinne, F.; Torres, A.; Porrini, E. Iohexol plasma clearance simplified by dried blood spot testing. *Nephrol. Dial. Transplant.* **2018**, *33*, 1597–1603. [CrossRef] [PubMed]

Journal of
Clinical Medicine

MDPI

Review

Compatibility of Post-Kidney Transplant Immunosuppression Therapy with Lactation

Gema Gomez-Casado [1,2], Juana Alonso-Titos [1,3], Ernesto Gonzalez-Mesa [1,4,5] and Almudena Ortega-Gomez [1,2,6,*]

1 Instituto de Investigación Biomédica de Málaga—IBIMA Plataforma BIONAND, University of Malaga, 29010 Malaga, Spain; gema.gomez@ibima.eu (G.G.-C.); juana12041988@hotmail.com (J.A.-T.); egonzalezmesa@uma.es (E.G.-M.)
2 Department of Endocrinology and Nutrition, Virgen de la Victoria University Hospital, 29010 Málaga, Spain
3 Nephrology Department, Regional University Hospital of Malaga, RICORS2040 (RD21/0005/0012-RD24/004/0026), 29010 Malaga, Spain
4 Department of Surgical Specialties, Biochemistry and Immunology, Faculty of Medicine, University of Malaga, 29010 Malaga, Spain
5 Department of Obstetrics and Gynecology Service, Regional University Hospital of Malaga, 29010 Malaga, Spain
6 CIBER Fisiopatologia Obesidad y Nutricion (CIBEROBN), Instituto de Salud Carlos III, 28029 Madrid, Spain
* Correspondence: almudena.ortega@ibima.eu

Abstract: Breastfeeding after kidney transplantation remains a complex and underexplored topic, primarily due to concerns regarding the safety of immunosuppressive therapies during lactation. Individuals who have received kidney transplants face a higher likelihood of delivering preterm infants and giving birth to babies with a low birth weight when compared with the general population. In this context, breastfeeding is increasingly important because of its advantages for preterm infants. Despite the well-established benefits of breastfeeding for both the mother and infant, the traditional recommendation has been to avoid nursing due to potential drug transmission through breast milk. However, emerging evidence suggests that certain immunosuppressants may be compatible with breastfeeding, challenging long-standing clinical guidelines. In this review, we examine the current literature on the pharmacokinetics, safety profiles, and clinical outcomes associated with key immunosuppressive agents, including cyclosporine, tacrolimus, everolimus, azathioprine, corticosteroids, and belatacept. Our work highlights that all published reports to date on the studied treatments indicate that the amount of the drug reaching breast milk is considered safe for the child's health. These conclusions, however, are derived from very short-term measurements and small numbers of patients. Therefore, we emphasize the need to design structured prospective studies to assess safety in the medium and long term. Our review aims to equip clinicians with the most up-to-date evidence on this topic, enabling them to make informed decisions regarding the compatibility of post-kidney transplant treatments with breastfeeding.

Keywords: kidney transplant; immunosuppression therapy; lactation; breastfeeding

1. Introduction

Women within the reproductive age range (18–49 years) who suffer from end-stage renal disease (ESRD) experience fertility rates that are almost 10 times lower compared to their healthy peers. According to the National Transplant Registry (NTPR), the live birth rate among recipients is between 71% and 79%, while the UK Transplant Registry reports a live birth rate of 79% [1]. The live birth rate among allograft recipients is similar to that of the general population. The occurrence of preterm deliveries has been noted to reach between 40% and 60%, in contrast to the 5% to 15% seen in the general population, primarily resulting from complications involving the mother or fetus rather than spontaneous preterm labor [1]. Furthermore, they have a higher prevalence of low birth weight (42–46%) and intrauterine growth restriction (30–50%) [2,3]. Additionally, the incidence of miscarriage ranges from 11% to 26%, in contrast to the 8% to 9% observed in the general population [1,4]. The effects of a low and extremely low birth weight on the fetus are significant, encompassing a range of neurological, endocrine, cardiac, and renal issues [5]. Research on the developmental outcomes in children born to transplant recipients is scarce. Data from the National Transplantation Pregnancy Registry (NTPR), based in the US, are limited but indicate that developmental delays have been observed in as many as 26% of children older than 5 years [1]. In situations of infertility, transplanted women often seek out assisted reproductive methods, with in vitro fertilization being the most common reproductive technique used. Case reports and population-based retrospective studies document favorable outcomes of pregnancies in transplanted mothers following induction medication treatment or in vitro fertilization [6].

Breastfeeding is the most effective way to support a child's growth and development. As a result, the World Health Organization recommends exclusive breastfeeding for the first 6 months and continued complementary breastfeeding for at least 3 years [7]. Children who are breastfed for more extended durations experience reduced rates of infectious diseases and deaths when compared to those breastfed for shorter times or not breastfed at all [8]. This difference persists into later life stages. Growing evidence suggests that breastfeeding also offers a safeguard against the risks of future overweight/obesity and diabetes [9,10]. For preterm infants, breastfeeding is crucial to their care and provides significant benefits for their growth and development. It helps reduce the risk of conditions such as necrotizing enterocolitis and late-onset sepsis [11,12], bronchopulmonary dysplasia [13], retinopathy of prematurity [14], and the likelihood of being readmitted to the hospital during the first year of life [15,16]. Additionally, it is linked to better neurodevelopmental results and enhanced cardiac performance [17]. Given the elevated rates of preterm births in pregnancies following kidney transplantation, breastfeeding is crucial for offering optimal support to infants born to mothers who have undergone transplantation.

2. Immunosuppression After Kidney Transplant

Graft damage and loss due to allograft rejection is a significant issue, with 7.0% of adult kidney transplant recipients experiencing acute rejection by 1 year [18]. There are two main types of rejection: T-cell-mediated rejection (TCMR) and antibody-mediated rejection (AMR). TCMR happens when donor-reactive CD4 and/or CD8 T cells infiltrate the allograft, causing inflammation and tissue damage [19]. On the other hand, AMR occurs when donor-specific antibodies bind to the allograft's endothelium, triggering the complement system and attracting leukocytes, which lead to graft damage [20]. The primary goal of immunosuppression is to enhance the longevity of the transplanted organ by avoiding rejection while reducing the side effects associated with treatment. After a transplant, immunosuppression consists of two stages: induction immunosuppression, given around the time of surgery to avert immediate rejection, and maintenance immunosuppression, provided on a continuous basis to support prolonged graft survival [21].

The administration of these immunosuppressants, which tend to be more effective with fewer adverse effects, has notably reduced both the mortality and morbidity rates. Immunosuppressive therapies include various agents, such as calcineurin inhibitors (e.g., cyclosporine-A and tacrolimus), antimetabolites (e.g., azathioprine), mTOR inhibitors (e.g., sirolimus and everolimus), and steroids. While these immunosuppressive drugs can lead to numerous side effects, such as hypertension, infections, and increased lipid levels, they are essential for preventing organ rejection. This highlights the necessity for personalized medication strategies [22]. Newer medications are key to enable more personalized treatment options. Selecting an appropriate immunosuppressive regimen should be personalized for each patient, considering the pharmacological properties of the drugs, their side effect profiles, potential interactions with other medications, as well as the patient's existing health conditions, risk of rejection, and current medication regimen. In this regard, evaluating how the treatment aligns with pregnancy and breastfeeding for individuals of reproductive age is essential.

3. Post-Kidney Transplant Immunosuppressive Treatments

Immunosuppression is generally accomplished by limiting the activity of lymphocytes. Over the decades, several treatment strategies have been employed to achieve this goal, including the use of calcineurin inhibitors, antiproliferative agents, mTOR inhibitors, and corticosteroids. These therapies, often used in combination, have evolved to enhance graft survival while minimizing adverse effects and the risk of infection. Continuous advancements in immunosuppressive regimens aim to refine this balance, improving long-term outcomes for kidney transplant recipients.

The arrival of calcineurin inhibitors (CNIs), specifically cyclosporine and tacrolimus, resulted in a reduction of rejection rates and enhanced short-term outcomes for both patients and grafts. However, prolonged use of these medications has been associated with kidney graft dysfunction, hypertension, hyperlipidemia, and diabetes mellitus. Sirolimus and everolimus, which are inhibitors of the mammalian target of rapamycin (mTOR), demonstrate effectiveness comparable to that of cyclosporine but come with side effects like delayed wound healing and hyperlipidemia [23–26]. Azathioprine is a pro-drug of 6-mercaptopurine (6-MP), a purine antagonist that inhibits leukocyte proliferation by interfering with nucleotide synthesis. Cytotoxic thioguanine nucleotides decrease the production of purine nucleotides via the de novo pathway by inhibiting amidotransferase enzymes and the interconversion of purine ribonucleotides. This mechanism is believed to cause the impact of azathioprine on the proliferation of leukocytes [27]. The corticosteroids utilized in transplantation medicine are primarily glucocorticoids, which are employed for their immune-modulating effects on the host's immune system to help reduce and minimize rejection. Glucocorticoids influence cells by attaching to the glucocorticoid receptor. The complex formed by the activated glucocorticoid receptor and glucocorticoid boosts the production of anti-inflammatory proteins in the nucleus (a process known as transactivation) and inhibits the synthesis of pro-inflammatory proteins in the cytosol by preventing the translocation of other transcription factors from the cytosol to the nucleus (transrepression) [28].

To mitigate the potential for nephrotoxicity associated with conventional therapies, newer treatments, including belatacept, a selective T-cell co-stimulation blocker, have been authorized in recent decades.

The mechanisms of action of the mentioned immunosuppressive drugs can be found in Table 1 and Figure 1.

Table 1. Most commonly used immunosuppressive drugs.

Group		Drug	Blocking Mechanisms
Immunophilin-binding treatments	Calcineurin inhibitors (CNIs)	Ciclosporin	Binds to cyclophilin, forming a complex that inhibits calcineurin, resulting in reduced cytokine production and diminished T-cell proliferation
		Tacrolimus	Binds to FK506-binding protein 12, forming a complex that inhibits calcineurin, thereby reducing cytokine production and T-cell proliferation
	mTOR inhibitors	Everolimus	Bind to FK506-binding protein 12, which, in turn, hinders mTOR, leading to a reduction in cytokine-induced T-cell proliferation
		Sirolimus	
Co-stimulation blockers	Cytotoxic T-lymphocyte-associated protein 4 (CTLA4)-Ig	Belatacept	Blocks co-stimulation of T-cell activity by CD28
Antimetabolites	Thiopurine	Azathioprine	Blocks purine production, leading to a decrease in T-cell growth
Corticoids	Glucocorticoids	Prednisone	Decrease the levels of circulating lymphocytes, monocytes, and eosinophils and suppress the production of cytokines
		Prednisolone	

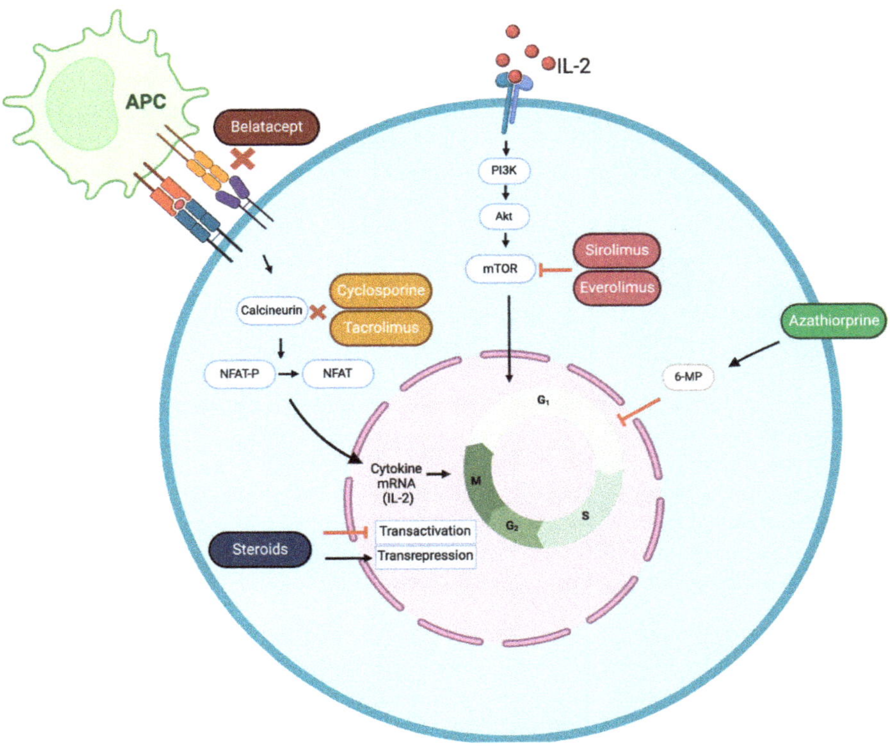

Figure 1. Mechanisms of action of most common immunosuppressive drugs: belatacept, cyclosporine, tacrolimus, sirolimus, everolimus, azathioprine, and steroids. APC: antigen-presenting cell.

4. Immunosuppressive Drugs and Breastfeeding

Individuals of reproductive age who have received transplants need guidance regarding the possible teratogenic effects associated with immunosuppressive therapy. Since pregnant women were traditionally excluded from trials involving immunosuppressants, safety information primarily comes from animal research and epidemiological studies derived from transplant pregnancy registries and specific case reports [29]. While acknowledging the potential risk of contact with immunosuppressants, it is important to consider that an infant's exposure to these substances through breastfeeding is less than that experienced in utero. The appropriateness of using immunosuppressive therapy during pregnancy has been examined in other sources, so it will not be addressed in this review in order to focus on breastfeeding [30–33]. Consequently, we explore the information available regarding the impact of maintenance immunosuppressive therapy in lactation.

To assess the exposure of children to medications taken by mothers through breast milk, several critical pharmacokinetic factors must be considered. On the one hand, it is important to understand how a medication transfers from the mother's bloodstream into breast milk and the anticipated concentration of the medication at specific times after administration. On the other hand, the expected absorption of the medication in the infant's gastrointestinal system and the amount of breast milk consumed are important factors. The transfer of medications from the maternal bloodstream to breast milk primarily occurs through passive diffusion. Similar to their transfer through the placenta, medications that are poorly protein bound, possess small molecular weights (less than 800 Dalton), and are highly lipophilic are more likely to be transferred into breast milk compared to larger and more hydrophilic substances [34].

The milk-to-plasma concentration ratio (M/P) of drugs is used to assess the amount of medication transferred to the breastfeeding infant. A M/P value of less than 1 indicates a low transfer of medication into breast milk. There is dependable information on M/P concentration ratios for only a limited number of drugs. The percentage of drug intake by infants through milk (adjusted for weight and time) is also utilized to examine how maternal drugs are distributed to infants. However, at this time, there is no suitable model available to forecast drug concentrations in human milk [34]. Likewise, a relative infant dose (RID), calculated as the weight-adjusted percentage of the maternal dose, which evaluates the projected infant dose based on the concentration of medication in breast milk and the volume ingested against the mother's dosage, of less than 10% is regarded as safe. Caution is advised for drugs that are excreted in amounts ranging from 10% to 25% of the maternal dose, while those excreted in quantities exceeding 25% are generally deemed unacceptable [35].

The availability of data regarding the safety of immunosuppressive treatment after transplantation is severely limited by the traditional recommendation to avoid breastfeeding during this therapy [36–38]. However, in recent decades, new research has surfaced that demonstrates the compatibility of certain immunosuppressive medications following organ transplants. In the following sections, we will delve into the available evidence regarding the most commonly used drugs, analyzing their mechanism of action, safety profiles, and potential interactions in post-transplant care.

4.1. Calcineurin Inhibitors

Calcineurin inhibitors (CNIs) are an essential class of immunosuppressive drugs commonly used to treat a range of autoimmune conditions. In addition to these applications, CNIs are vital in preventing organ rejection by providing crucial immunosuppression in solid organ transplantation. The most commonly used CNIs in post-transplant immunosuppressive therapy are cyclosporine and tacrolimus (Table 1). These drugs work by binding with high specificity and affinity to specific cytoplasmic receptors, collectively known as immunophilins, such as cyclophilin and FK-binding proteins. By inhibiting calcineurin, CNIs block a key signaling pathway that leads to the transcription of interleukin-2 and other important cytokines, like IL-4, interferon-γ (IFN-γ), and tumor necrosis factor-α (TNF-α). This pathway involves NFAT, a DNA-binding protein crucial for interleukin-2 gene transcription. In unstimulated T cells, NFAT consists of a subunit (NFATp) that interacts with Fos and Jun proteins in the nucleus of activated T cells [39]. The blockage of this route disrupts the activation, proliferation, and differentiation of T lymphocytes, which are integral to the immune response, thereby reducing the risk of rejection in transplant recipients and controlling autoimmune activity in affected individuals [40] (Figure 1). The enzyme CYP3A4, which is responsible for metabolizing both CNIs, shows an increase in its expression within the neonatal liver after birth. This upregulation leads to a reduced concentration of these drugs in the bloodstream of infants shortly after delivery [41].

4.1.1. Cyclosporine

In the majority of breastfed infants, cyclosporine is undetectable in the bloodstream. However, there have been instances where detectable blood levels were observed, even when both the milk concentration and the infant's calculated dose were relatively low. Cyclosporine levels exhibit significant variability across different case reports and series assessed. This variation is likely due to discrepancies in sampling times across studies and is probably influenced by the fat content of the milk at the time of collection. When maternal cyclosporine blood levels are within the typical range, a fully breastfed infant usually receives no more than 2% of the mother's weight-adjusted dose or the pediatric transplantation maintenance dose and often less than 1% [42]. There have been no reported cases of adverse effects on infants' growth, development, or kidney function. As a result, guidelines from the United States and Europe, along with the National Transplantation Pregnancy Registry and other experts, deem the use of cyclosporine during breastfeeding to be acceptable [43,44]. However, it is important to note that comprehensive follow-up examinations may not have always been conducted or documented.

We have identified 14 reports, spanning from 1983 to 2022, that examine the transfer of cyclosporine into breast milk and its short-term effects on infants. The amount of cyclosporine detected in breast milk in these studies varied between 0.4 μg/mL and 564 μg/mL, and the maternal weight-adjusted dose ranged between 0.01% and 2.1%, far below the limit of 10% to be considered safe [35]. When reported, no clinical adverse effects were found in the infants. However, most of these studies are based on a single patient and are limited to short-term follow-up, with little consistency between articles.

In addition to case reports, studies conducted on animals have demonstrated the harmless effects of cyclosporin during lactation. One particular study found that although the levels of cyclosporin in mother rats were quite high, the cyclosporin levels in the pups from the 21-day treatment group were non-existent. Renal histomorphometric comparisons between the study pups and the control pups showed no significant differences in either age group. However, when examining renal function parameters, significant distinctions were observed between the study and control pups in the infancy category: pups in the 21-day treatment group exhibited a notably lower urine volume, proteinuria, FE (Na), and urinary NAG/creatinine ratio. Although the glomerular filtration rate was lower in the 21-day treatment group, this difference was not statistically significant, and there were no significant variations in serum creatinine levels [45]. A compilation of human studies testing the effect of cyclosporin on breastfeeding is detailed in Table 2.

4.1.2. Tacrolimus

Tacrolimus, previously known as FK506, is a macrolide antibiotic that has immunosuppressive capabilities. While it is structurally different from cyclosporin, its mechanism of action is comparable. Tacrolimus exerts its primary effects by disrupting gene expression in target cells. It binds to an immunophilin called FK506 binding protein (FKBP), forming a complex that interferes with calcineurin phosphatase. This action inhibits calcium-dependent processes, including interleukin-2 gene transcription, the activation of nitric oxide synthase, cell degranulation, and apoptosis. Tacrolimus also amplifies the effects of glucocorticoids and progesterone by binding to FKBPs in the hormone receptor complex, preventing their degradation. The drug may increase the expression of the TGF-β gene, similar to cyclosporine. Tacrolimus inhibits T-cell proliferation in response to T-cell receptor ligation and appears to preferentially suppress type 1 T helper cells over type 2 T helper cells. B-cell growth and antibody production are indirectly affected by the suppression of T-cell-derived growth factors essential for these activities. Antigen presentation appears to remain unaffected. The molecular mechanisms influenced by tacrolimus are still being explored [39].

Twelve studies have been found on tacrolimus, its transfer to breast milk, and its effect on children. The amount of drug found in breast milk ranged between 0.5 μg/mL and 3.8 μg/mL, while the infant blood drug levels varied between 0.2 μg/L and 3.2 μg/L. In any case, the lowest maternal weight-adjusted dose value was 0.23%, and the highest was 0.5%, with both of them considered safe. The infants were reported to grow and develop normally, physically and neurologically, with no signs of metabolic disorders or significant infections. Although in this case there are several reports studying a group of patients ranging from 4 to 14, the results should be interpreted with caution due to the disparity between studies. Table 2 provides a summary of the studies examining the impact of tacrolimus on breastfeeding.

4.2. Thiopurine Drugs (Antimetabolites)

Thiopurine medications are purine antimetabolites commonly utilized in treating acute lymphoblastic leukemia, autoimmune conditions (such as Crohn's disease and rheumatoid arthritis), and for patients who have undergone organ transplants. As pro-drugs that are inactive in their initial form, 6-mercaptopurine (6-MP), 6-thioguanine (6-TG), and azathioprine must undergo intracellular activation, which is facilitated by various enzymes, in order to produce their cytotoxic effects [46].

Azathioprine

Azathioprine is a pro-drug of 6-MP that was originally investigated as a chemotherapeutic drug for the treatment of leukemia [28]. 6-MP acts as a purine antagonist, hindering the proliferation of leukocytes by disrupting nucleotide synthesis (Figure 1). Azathioprine has a superior therapeutic index compared to 6-MP, which has resulted in azathioprine playing a more prominent role in the treatment options for managing systemic autoimmune diseases [47]. There have been rare reports of hyperprolactinemia and galactorrhea occurring with normal prolactin levels [48,49]. However, expert guidelines from North America and Europe, along with the US-based NTPR and other specialists, regard azathioprine as a suitable option for use while breastfeeding [50–52]. Thirteen studies have been identified reporting on azathioprine medication during breastfeeding, with a study group size between 1 and 34 patients. When reported, the levels of azathioprine or 6-MP measured in breast milk across these studies ranged from 1.2 to 50 μg/mL, being measured at different time points. High drug levels were undetected in the infant's blood, and the calculated maternal weight-adjusted dose ranged between 0.05 and 1%, which is, in principle, considered safe.

One infant was reported to have a borderline low neutrophil count but a normal white cell count. Otherwise, no adverse effects were encountered in the infants, who showed normal growth, normal mental and physical development, and no above-average infection incidence. In Table 2, a summary of reports on the impact of azathioprine on breastfeeding is presented.

Table 2. Reports on compatibility of most commonly used immunosuppressive drugs with breastfeeding.

Immuno-suppressive Agent	Dose	Subject Group	Drug Levels in Breast Milk	Effects on the Infant	Year	Reference
Cyclosporine	450 mg/day during pregnancy	1	101, 109, and 263 μg/L in breastmilk on days 2, 3, and 4 postpartum	Not specified.	1983	[53]
	325 mg 2 h before the onset of labor	1	16 μg/L	Undetectable (<3 μg//L) cyclosporine blood levels.	1985	[54]
	225 mg/day	1	Not reported	Estimated intake of 6 μg/kg daily (0.01% maternal weight-adjusted dose); the infant remained healthy and normal.	1995	[55]
	3 mg/kg twice daily	1	596 μg/L 5 weeks postpartum; the infant would receive less than 0.1 mg/kg per day or no more than 1.7% of the maternal weight-adjusted dose	At 5 weeks of age, normal renal function and a blood cyclosporin concentration below 3 μg/L; estimated levels taken through milk (150 mL/Kg/day) < 0.1 mg/kg of cyclosporin.	1997	[56]
	Not reported	5	50 to 227 ng/mL	All infants had levels below the detection limit of 30 ng/mL. Breastfed infants of mothers on cyclosporine received less than 300 μg/day, with absorption amounts being undetectable. No nephrotoxic effects or other side effects were observed.	1998	[57]
		1	25 to 120 μg/L			
		1	87 to 440 μg/L			
	300 mg twice daily	1	79 to 286 μg/L on three separate occasions over a 10-week period	The breast milk/maternal blood level ratio was 84%, but the infant had undetectable levels. The infant grew and developed normally.	2001	[58]
	5.3 mg/kg per day	1	403 μg/L	The estimated dose the infant would ingest through breast milk was 0.06 mg/kg/day (1.1% of the weight-adjusted maternal dose), 1% of the therapeutic dose on a weight basis.	2003	[59]
	225 mg/day	1	465 μg/L in foremilk and 564 μg/L in hindmilk	The estimated dose the infant would ingest through breast milk was 0.08 mg/kg/day (2.1% of the weight-adjusted maternal dose). The cyclosporine concentration in the infant's blood was below the detection limit of 25 μg/L.		
	250 mg/day	1	97.6 μg/L	The estimated dose the infant would ingest through breast milk was 0.01 mg/kg per day (0.2% of the weight-adjusted maternal dose). Cyclosporine levels in the infant's blood were below the detection limit.		
	250 mg/day	1	117.7 μg/L ranged from 75 to 150 μg/L	The infant received a dose of 0.4% of the weight-adjusted maternal dose. The infant's blood concentration was below the detection limit of 25 μg/L.		
	150 mg twice daily	1	Two points measurement on day 8 yielded 84 and 144 μg/L	Infant exposure is estimated to be 0.5% of the maternal weight-adjusted dose. Breastfeeding continued without any adverse effects observed.		

Table 2. *Cont.*

Immuno-suppressive Agent	Dose	Subject Group	Drug Levels in Breast Milk	Effects on the Infant	Year	Reference
Cyclosporine	100 mg in the morning and 75 mg in the evening	1	46 μg/L	The estimated dose the infant would ingest through breast milk was 0.007 mg/kg, or 0.33% of the weight-adjusted maternal dose. The infant's blood levels were undetectable (<10 μg/L), and no apparent clinical adverse effects from cyclosporine were observed.	2011	[60]
	200 mg/day	1	Not reported	The infant's serum cyclosporine level was undetectable (with an assay lower limit of 15 mg/L). The mother continued breastfeeding for 5 months, during which her infant remained healthy and had normal renal function.	2011	[61]
	120 mg/day	1		The infant's serum cyclosporine level was undetectable, with a lower assay limit of 15 mg/L.		
	5 mg/kg	1	Not reported	The infant's serum cyclosporine concentrations after the morning feed were consistently undetectable (<30 μg/L).	2011	[62]
	200 mg/day	1	128 μg/L, 200 μg/L, and 364 μg/L on days 10, 30, and 50 after morning dose: on day 40, before her morning dose, was 207 μg/L	By 12 months of age, the infant was developing normally and showed no noticeable adverse effects from the drug in the breast milk.	2014	[63]
	1.5 mg/kg/day	1	15.5 μg/L in colostrum	In the newborn, cyclosporine disappeared within 2 days. No immediate complications were observed with this pregnancy.	2016	[64]
	200 mg/day	7	22.4 μg/L	The mean cyclosporine concentration in the colostrum was 22.40 ± 9.43 μg/L, with an estimated mean daily dose of 1049.22 ± 397.41 ng/kg/24 h. The average daily infant dosage was estimated to be 1.05 μg/kg.	2020	[65]
	125 mg in the morning and 100 mg at night, totaling 3 mg/kg/day	1	0.443 μg/L to 5.3 μg/L	At the three-month follow-up, both twin infants were growing and developing normally, with no adverse effects observed.	2022	[66]
Tacrolimus	3 mg/day	1	0.57 μg//L one hour after the dose	The average amount of tacrolimus that neonates would ingest through maternal milk was 151.4 ng/kg/24 h. The peak tacrolimus concentration in colostrum was observed 8 h after an oral dose, reaching 3.219 ng/mL. The low concentrations of tacrolimus in colostrum indicate that the neonates would ingest only trace amounts of the drug. The infant was developing normally, both physically and neurologically.	2003	[67]
	2 mg twice daily	1	Average 1.8 μg/L, with a milk-to-blood ratio of 0.23	The baby ingested about 0.5% of the maternal weight-adjusted dose. The authors calculated that an exclusively breastfed infant would receive a daily dose of 0.27 μg/kg, which is approximately 0.5% of the maternal weight-adjusted dose and less than 0.2% of the pediatric dose for organ transplant rejection.	2006	[68]
	Not reported	6	0.3 to 1.9 μg/L, with average 1.7 μg/L	Normal prenatal growth for the gestational age and postnatal growth for the infant's postpartum age.	2010	[69]
	9.6 mg/day (range from 4.5 to 15 mg/day)	4	Not reported	Whole-blood drug concentrations between day 15 and day 27 after delivery were undetectable, with a lower limit of detection of <1.9 μg/L.	2012	[70]

Table 2. *Cont.*

Immuno-suppressive Agent	Dose	Subject Group	Drug Levels in Breast Milk	Effects on the Infant	Year	Reference
Tacrolimus	6 mg twice daily	1	Not reported	Infant's drug blood level was less than 1 µg/L.	2012	[71]
	Dose not specified, but assumed to be 6 mg/day	14	0.8 µg//L average (range 0.1 to 1.6 µg//L)	All infants experienced a 15% daily decline in tacrolimus levels. The maximum estimated absorption from breast milk was 0.23% of the maternal dose (weight-adjusted). The highest dosage an exclusively breastfed infant would receive is 0.56 µg/day, which is equivalent to 0.23% of the maternal weight-adjusted dose.	2013	[72]
	Average 7.5 mg/day	8	Average 0.93 ng/mL	Infants were exposed to less than 0.3% of the mother's weight-adjusted tacrolimus dose through breast milk. With such low levels of neonatal drug exposure, it is considered unlikely to pose any health risk to the breastfeeding infant.	2013	[73]
	4 to 14 mg/day	14	Average 3.2 µg/L	The average amount of tacrolimus ingested by neonates through maternal milk was 151.4 ng/kg/24 h. The highest concentration was observed 8 h after an oral dose, reaching 3.219 ng/mL. The low concentrations of tacrolimus indicate that neonates are exposed to only trace amounts of the drug.	2013	[74]
	3 mg daily	2	Not reported	At 1 hour after breastfeeding, the first infant's blood drug level was 0.2 µg/L at 10 days of age, while the second infant's level was 0.5 µg/L at 7 days of age.	2014	[75]
	3.2 mg/day (range 2 to 5.5 mg)	13	The median levels were 3 µg/L at trough, 3.8 µg/L at 2 h, and 3.7 µg/L at 12 h	The relative infant dose in breastfed infants was less than 1%, and the drug levels in the infant's blood were below detectable limits.	2018	[76]
	1.5 mg twice daily	1	At 4 days postpartum, the milk level was 1.1 µg/L; at 21 days postpartum, the milk levels were 1.4 µg/L at the time of the morning dose, 1.3 µg/L 4 h after the dose, 1.6 µg/L 8 h after the dose, and 1.4 µg/L 12 h after the dose	The breast milk-to-maternal blood ratio ranged from 0.40 to 0.64. Tacrolimus was undetectable in the neonate three weeks after birth. The authors estimated that a fully breastfed infant would receive 0.4% of the mother's weight-adjusted dose.	2021	[77]
	Not reported	1	0.5 µg/L	The infant showed normal weight gain and motor development, with no indications of metabolic disorders or significant infections. The child's exposure to the drug was extremely low, with the blood concentration approximately 90 times lower than the mother's.	2024	[78]
Everolimus	2 mg daily during pregnancy	1	Undetectable levels (<0.5 µg/L) in colostrum 1 day postpartum	Estimated elimination half-life of everolimus was estimated at 86 h in the newborn.	2016	[64]
	0.5 mg/day	1	Highest level was 66 ng/L	The estimated infant dose of the drug was 4.224 ng/kg/24 h, which accounted for 0.38% of the mother's dose.	2017	[79]

Table 2. *Cont.*

Immuno-suppressive Agent	Dose	Subject Group	Drug Levels in Breast Milk	Effects on the Infant	Year	Reference
Azathioprine	75 mg/day	1	Peak colostrum levels (2 days postpartum) 2 and 8 h after oral dose, being 3.4 and 4.5 μg/L, respectively	The milk levels in these two mothers were equivalent to 0.05% and 0.6% of the maternal weight-adjusted doses, respectively. Infant serum levels were not assessed.	1982	[80]
	25 mg oral dose	1	Peak 6-MP milk level of 18 μg/L occurred 2 h after oral dose (7 days postpartum)			
	Not reported	2	Not reported	The infants exhibited normal blood cell counts, no increase in infections, and an above-average growth rate.	2008	[81]
	100 mg/day	1	6-MP was not detected five weeks after birth	With a detection limit of 5 μg/L, the infant would have ingested a maximum of 0.09% of the mother's weight-adjusted dose. The child remained healthy and breastfed for 12 months.	1995	[55]
	1.2 to 2.1 mg/kg/day	4	Not reported	At 3 to 3.5 months of age, none of the infants had detectable blood levels of 6-TGNs and 6-MP.	2006	[82]
	100 mg/day	2	In 5 and 6 milk samples of each subject collected over a 24 h period, 6-MP was undetectable (<5 μg/L)	The absolute relative infant dose would have been under 0.09% of the maternal weight-adjusted dose, and no adverse effects were observed in the infants.	2006	[83]
	75 mg/day	1	Not reported	At the 1-month follow-up, the growth and development of the breastfeeding infant were reported as normal.		
	50 mg/day	1	Not reported	No adverse effects were observed in this child during the 2-month follow-up.		
	75 to 150 mg/day	10	Only one woman on 100 mg/day of azathioprine had detectable 6-MP in her milk; on day 28 postpartum, milk concentrations were 1.2 μg/L at 3 h and 7.6 μg/L at 6 h after the dose; no 6-MP was found in any of the other 29 milk samples	6-MP and 6-TGN were undetectable in the neonatal blood. None of the ten neonates showed clinical or hematological signs of immunosuppression during the first 28 days postpartum. One infant had a slightly low neutrophil count, but the overall white cell count remained normal.	2007	[84]
	75–200 mg/day	8	Peak 6-MP concentrations in milk were observed within the first 4 h after the dose, ranging from 2 to 50 μg/L	The estimated infant intake was less than 0.008 mg/kg body weight per 24 h, representing less than 1% of the maternal weight-adjusted dose.	2008	[85]
	100 mg (1.4 mg/kg) daily	1	Not reported	At both 8-days and 3-months postpartum, 6-TGNs were undetectable in the infant's blood. Over the 6-month follow-up period, the child thrived and experienced no infections.	2009	[86]
	Median dose 150 mg/day (range 100 to 250 mg/day)	11	Not reported	There were no differences in mental or physical development between the two groups of infants, nor was there any variation in the incidence of other infections between the groups.	2011	[87]
	1.93 mg/Kg (AZA), 0.94–1.32 mg/Kg (6-MP)	Mothers taking either azathioprine (n = 28) or 6-MP (n = 2)	Not reported	In this cohort, nine infants were breastfed for an average of 7 months (ranging from 3 to 13 months). No statistically significant differences were observed between breastfed and formula-fed infants across any of the 12 survey domains.	2013	[88]

Table 2. *Cont.*

Immuno-suppressive Agent	Dose	Subject Group	Drug Levels in Breast Milk	Effects on the Infant	Year	Reference
Prednisone	Single 10 mg oral dose	1	28.3 μg/L	N.A.	1975	[89]
	Single 20 mg oral dose	1	102 μg/L	N.A.	1981	[90]
	10 to 80 mg/day	6	Milk concentrations were 5% to 25% of those in serum.	At a daily dose of 80 mg of prednisolone, the infant would consume less than 0.1% of that dose, which is equivalent to less than 10% of the infant's natural cortisol production.	1985	[91]
	Single 50 mg (intravenous dose)	3	Only 0.025% of the prednisolone dose (ranging from 0.010% to 0.049%) was found in the milk	N.A.	1993	[92]
	2 mg every 12 h	1	Prednisone levels in milk were undetectable (<4 μg/L) after 12 h, while prednisolone levels were undetectable after 6 h	The weight-adjusted infant dosages were 0.58% and 0.35% of the maternal prednisone dose and 0.18% and 0.09% of the maternal prednisolone dose.	2019	[93]
	15 mg every 24 h	1				
Belatacept	10 mg/kg monthly	1	Not reported	Normal growth and cognitive development.	2020	[94]
	Not reported	5	Not reported	No reports of problems breastfeeding or issues in the children.	2023	[95]

(6-MP: 6-mercaptopurine; 6-TGNs: 6-thioguanine nucleosides; AZA: azathioprine; N.A.: non-applicable).

4.3. mTOR Inhibitors

Mammalian target of rapamycin (mTOR) inhibitors are a class of drugs that disrupt the complex mTOR signaling pathway, thereby reducing T-cell growth and the alloimmune reaction. Two mTOR inhibitors have been approved and are used in kidney transplantation: sirolimus and everolimus. These drugs interact with immunophillins needed to inhibit cell growth and proliferation (Table 1). The primary trigger for the proliferation of activated T cells in this instance is IL-2. The IL-2 receptor is activated by IL-2 produced in an autocrine manner, which propagates the proliferation signal through PIK3 and Akt pathways. The inhibition of mTOR interferes with the metabolic status and differentiation of activated T cells, limiting their proliferation [96] (Figure 1). Because of the nephrotoxic effects associated with calcineurin inhibitors, mTOR inhibitors have emerged as immunosuppressive agents for use after transplantation.

4.3.1. Sirolimus

Sirolimus has a high molecular weight (914.2), which may limit its transfer into breast milk, along with its low oral bioavailability. However, it has a long half-life of around 60 h in adults, and prescribing information notes that only trace amounts were detected in the milk of lactating rats [97].

Information regarding breastfeeding in human patients taking sirolimus is scarce, with only one case report available about a kidney–pancreas recipient. Unfortunately, this report lacks any details about the levels of the medication in both maternal and infant plasma, as well as in breast milk [72]. Therefore, further research on this drug is needed to begin analyzing its compatibility with breastfeeding.

4.3.2. Everolimus

Similar to sirolimus, everolimus has a high molecular weight of 958 and a low oral bioavailability. While its half-life of 30 h is relatively long, it is shorter than that of sirolimus [97]. Currently, two case reports have examined everolimus levels in the breast milk of transplant recipients after childbirth, although neither patient elected to breastfeed. In one of them, a female transplanted patient received everolimus (2 mg/day) during pregnancy and postpartum. Although she did not breastfeed, colostrum collected one day after delivery showed undetectable everolimus levels. Serial plasma measurements indicated an estimated everolimus elimination half-life of 86 h in the newborn [64]. The second study on a transplant recipient receiving everolimus (0.5 mg) during pregnancy and postpartum reported a pre-dose everolimus level of 33 ng/L, peaking at 66 ng/L four hours post-dose. Levels at 2, 6, 8, and 12 h post-dose ranged from 45 to 51 ng/L, and the estimated dose for infants was calculated to be 4.22 ng/kg/24 h, representing 0.38% of the dose given to the mother [79] (Table 2).

4.4. *Corticosteroids*

Corticosteroids encompass both the primary endogenous glucocorticoid, cortisol, and synthetic therapeutic agents like prednisone and methylprednisolone. In transplantation medicine, glucocorticoids are the most commonly used corticosteroids due to their immunomodulatory properties. These compounds exert their effects by binding to the glucocorticoid receptor, forming a complex that regulates gene expression. This complex enhances the production of anti-inflammatory proteins within the nucleus (transactivation) while simultaneously suppressing pro-inflammatory protein expression in the cytosol by preventing the migration of transcription factors into the nucleus (transrepression) [28] (Figure 1).

No negative effects have been observed in breastfeeding infants when mothers use any corticosteroid while nursing. While it is frequently advised to refrain from breastfeeding for four hours after taking a dose, this practice might be unnecessary as the levels of prednisone in breast milk are quite low [98]. Most commonly used corticosteroid in kidney transplant regimens is prednisone.

The reports found on the use of prednisone during breastfeeding can be seen in Table 2. These articles' study patient groups ranged from 1 to 6 individuals, and the levels of prednisone found in breastmilk ranged from undetectable (<4 µg/L) to 102 µg/L. Only 2 of these studies reported levels of prednisone in the infant's blood, and the weight-adjusted dosages were between 0.1 and 0.58%, which is, in principle, considered safe. Table 2 shows a summary of these studies.

The use of steroids during pregnancy carries the risk of developing steroid-induced diabetes mellitus, characterized by an unusual rise in blood sugar levels linked to the administration of glucocorticoids, which may require careful monitoring and management to minimize potential complications for both the mother and the baby. Although limited documentation exists on this topic, this factor should be taken into account when evaluating the choices regarding corticosteroid therapy.

4.5. *Belatacept*

As an alternative to more traditional treatments, to prevent rejection and avoid their long-term side effects, new drugs to block T-cell activation have been recently developed. Belatacept is a protein resulting from combining the Fc region of immunoglobulin IgG1 and the extracellular domain of CTLA-4, therefore termed (CTLA-4)-Ig. To activate a T cell and elicit an immune response, the antigen-presenting cell must provide two types of signals to the T cell. One involves the major histocompatibility complex (MHC) in conjunction with the antigen, while the other signal is provided by the CD80 or CD86 molecule. Belatacept interacts the CD80 and CD86 molecules, resulting in the inhibition of the second signal from CD28 [99] (Figure 1). Belatacept has been the last immunosuppressive drug to be approved by American and European agencies since 2012 [100,101] and has shown significant improvement in renal function following kidney transplantation, as compared to CNIs [102]. Due to its recent approval, the availability of studies on belatacept and breastfeeding are limited to two studies, in which transplanted mothers breastfed their babies while maintaining the belatacept treatment, with normal growth and cognitive infant development reported [94,95] (Table 2).

The long-term management of maintenance immunosuppression in kidney transplant recipients is still complicated. While CNIs remain the preferred treatment option, their nephrotoxicity necessitates continuous evaluation and the search for alternatives. Current options include belatacept or mTOR inhibitors. While treatment with belatacept results in better kidney function at the 7-year evaluation compared to CNIs, it presents high initial rejection rates.

5. Additional Considerations

In addition to the immunosuppressive therapies discussed in this text, kidney transplantation often requires additional treatments to ensure compatibility with the graft and the patient's survival. Consequently, prior to deciding about breastfeeding, it is crucial to assess the compatibility of these substances. Some examples are antihypertensive medication such as Angiotensin-Converting Enzyme Inhibitors (ACEIs)/Angiotensin II Receptor Blockers (ARBs), Calcium Channel Blockers (CCBs), and Sodium–Glucose Transport Protein 2 Inhibitors (SGLT2i); lipid-lowering agents like statins, antibiotics, and Erythropoiesis-Stimulating Agents (ESAs); and gastrointestinal protective drugs such as proton pump inhibitors (PPIs) or H2 blockers. A promising option is the combination of a low dose of tacrolimus with an Angiotensin-Converting Enzyme Inhibitor (ACEi)/Angiotensin II Receptor 1 Blocker (ARB) treatment to achieve adequate immunosuppression and protection against chronic scarring [103]. However, the compatibility of these agents with breastfeeding should be clinically evaluated within the context of the patient's overall treatment plan.

The immunosuppressive treatments explained in this review focus on TCMR; however, AMR is a major contributor to late graft loss in kidney transplant recipients. Patients with high levels of donor-specific antibodies are at a higher risk of AMR and, consequently, graft loss [104]. Plasmapheresis, also known as plasma exchange, is the primary treatment used in kidney transplantation to remove donor-specific antibodies. Regarding its compatibility with lactation, most of the available evidence comes from plasma-exchange treatments during pregnancy in thrombotic microangiopathies, lipid disorders, and a variety of autoimmune diseases [105]. The use of plasmapheresis during pregnancy is primarily based on individual case reports, as there is a lack of high-quality studies and conclusive evidence-based guidelines. Therefore, scientific evidence on the compatibility of plasma-exchange therapy with breastfeeding in kidney transplantation is too limited to be properly assessed.

6. Discussion

In addition to the decrease in fertility rates, women who have undergone transplantation face an increased risk of preterm births, while babies born to these mothers often have low birth weights and may experience intrauterine growth restriction [2,3]. Given the established significance of breastfeeding in these situations, it is crucial to ensure that these infants have access to maternal milk. Due to the traditional discouragement of breastfeeding among transplanted mothers, there is limited information on the compatibility of certain immunosuppressant medications with lactation. Nonetheless, the latest guidelines increasingly highlight the compatibility of post-transplant treatment with breastfeeding, drafting a promising and optimistic outlook.

In 2013, Thiagarajan et al. released guidelines concerning breastfeeding after transplantation, organized around three specific scenarios. First, breastfeeding should be avoided when medications with known harmful effects are being used. Second, breastfeeding might either continue or be temporarily halted depending on the newborn's serum levels of drugs that are typically regarded as safe at low concentrations, like cyclosporine, tacrolimus, corticosteroids, and azathioprine. Third, careful consideration is necessary when using medications with uncertain safety profiles, including mTOR inhibitors. These guidelines highlighted the need to find a balance between the health outcomes of the mother and infant while managing immunosuppressive therapies after transplantation during lactation [44]. Although more than a decade has passed since these recommendations, information regarding the levels of mTOR inhibitors in breast milk is still limited, underscoring the necessity for conducting further research on this topic. Furthermore, there appears to be a level of inconsistency in the existing studies concerning the presence of post-transplant immunosuppressive medications in breast milk, likely due to the unclear timing of sample collection in relation to maternal dosing and variations in assay methods.

Earlier pediatric guidelines have stated that some medications are present in human milk only in minimal amounts, and their mere presence does not automatically imply a risk to the infant. As a result, healthcare professionals are encouraged to consider multiple factors when providing guidance to those who require medication during breastfeeding [51].

Although there are currently reports with data on the subject, the compatibility of immunosuppressive drugs with lactation remains an area of limited research. The available reports are scarce and involve small patient cohorts, making it difficult to draw definitive conclusions. While low drug transfer to breast milk and minimal infant exposure have been reported, there is significant variability among studies. Additionally, follow-up periods are often short, ranging from 1 to 3 months in most cases, with only a few extending to 12–18 months. This limited timeframe restricts the ability to assess potential long-term effects in infants. Despite the theoretical safety suggested by low drug levels in breast milk, the absence of robust, long-term data prevents definitive recommendations for now. More extensive, well-designed studies with larger sample sizes and longer follow-up are necessary to evaluate the true impact of immunosuppressive therapy during lactation. Until then, the decision to breastfeed while on these medications should be individualized, weighing potential benefits against unknown risks.

When seeking the optimal approach to reconcile the use of immunosuppressant medications with lactation, adjusting the timing of drug administration and breastfeeding may be crucial. This can help minimize the exposure of the infant to the medications while ensuring the mother's health is maintained. Strategies such as coordinating the timing of medication doses to occur immediately after a breastfeeding session or during periods when the infant will not be nursing for a longer time could be key to achieving both effective treatment and safe breastfeeding.

7. Conclusions and Future Directions

Based on the currently available evidence, it can be concluded that the indications suggest that breastfeeding may be compatible with the use of the studied medications. However, several limitations must be considered: the small sample sizes, the lack of methodological consistency across studies, and the absence of long-term follow-up. Furthermore, to aid in drawing conclusions about each medication, this review has examined them separately. Nevertheless, treatments following a kidney transplant generally consist of combinations of them.

Regarding the need to generate more consistent and reliable scientific evidence, it is essential to design prospective studies with matched control groups and, if possible, multicenter collaborations. Sample analysis should be scheduled from the first month (short term), continuing through 6–18 months (mid-term), and ideally extending follow-up to at least 5 years (long term). This framework is crucial to effectively monitor cognitive and growth development, immune response, allergy development, as well as metabolic and neurological health in infants exposed to maternal medication through breastfeeding.

Future clinical guidelines should focus on maintaining the therapeutic effect in the mother while minimizing drug exposure in the infant. To achieve this, several factors need to be taken into account: the dosage and frequency of the treatment, its pharmacokinetics, the infant's health status, and the implementation of a breastfeeding schedule that maximizes the time interval between medication intake and nursing sessions. Overall, the prevailing perspective is that adjusting immunosuppressive dosages, in conjunction with oversight from a high-risk obstetrician, is crucial for ensuring safe breastfeeding [106].

In conclusion, while significant progress has been made in recent decades, much work remains to be conducted. The continuous updating of best practices and guidelines, incorporating the latest research on the topic, is essential for providing optimal care. Achieving a balance between the health benefits for both the mother and child while minimizing potential risks to the infant is key to advancing this area of clinical practice.

Author Contributions: Conceptualization, A.O.-G. and E.G.-M. Funding acquisition, A.O.-G. Literature review, G.G.-C. and J.A.-T. Writing—original draft, G.G.-C. and J.A.-T. Writing—review and editing, A.O.-G. and E.G.-M. All authors have read and agreed to the published version of the manuscript.

Funding: This study was supported by the research project PI22/01813, funded by the Instituto de Salud Carlos III (ISCIII) and co-funded by the European Union, and by the Research Project ProyExcel_00962, from Consejería de Universidad, Investigación e Innovación de Andalucía to A.O.-G. and E.G.-M. G.G.-C. is supported by a PFIS contract (FI23/00104), and A.O-G holds a Miguel Servet position (CP20/0060), both from ISCIII and co-funded by the European Union.

Conflicts of Interest: The authors declare no conflicts of interest.

Abbreviations

The following abbreviations are used in this manuscript:

ESRD	End-stage renal disease
NTPR	National Transplant Registry
AMR	Antibody-mediated rejection
TCMR	T-cell mediated rejection
M/P	Milk-to-plasma concentration ratio of drugs
RID	Relative infant dose
CNIs	Calcineurin inhibitors
6-MP	6-mercaptopurine
6-TG	6-thioguanine
mTOR	mammalian target Of rapamycin

References

1. Armenti, V.T.; Daller, J.A.; Constantinescu, S.; Silva, P.; Radomski, J.S.; Moritz, M.J.; Gaughan, W.J.; McGrory, C.H.; Coscia, L.A. CT06 Chapter 4: Report from the National Transplantation Pregnancy Registry: Outcomes of Pregnancy After Transplantation. *Clin. Transpl.* **2006**, *4*, 57–70.
2. Sgro, M.D.; Barozzino, T.; Mirghani, H.M.; Sermer, M.; Moscato, L.; Akoury, H.; Koren, G.; Chitayat, D.A. Pregnancy outcome post renal transplantation. *Teratology* **2002**, *65*, 5–9. [CrossRef]
3. Colon, M.d.M.; Hibbard, J.U. Obstetric considerations in the management of pregnancy in kidney transplant recipients. *Adv. Chronic Kidney Dis.* **2007**, *14*, 168–177. [CrossRef]
4. Sibanda, N.; Briggs, J.D.; Davison, J.M.; Johnson, R.J.; Rudge, C.J. Pregnancy after organ transplantation: A report from the UK transplant pregnancy registry. *Transplantation* **2007**, *83*, 1301–1307. [CrossRef] [PubMed]
5. McKay, D.B.; Josephson, M.A. Pregnancy after Kidney Transplantation. *Clin. J. Am. Soc. Nephrol.* **2008**, *3* (Suppl. S2), S117–S125. [CrossRef] [PubMed]
6. Caretto, A.; Caldara, R.; Castiglioni, M.T.; Scavini, M.; Secchi, A. Pregnancy after pancreas-kidney transplantation. *J. Nephrol.* **2020**, *33*, 1009–1018. [CrossRef]
7. WHO. Protecting, Promoting and Supporting Breastfeeding in Facilities Providing Maternity and Newborn Services. 2017. Available online: https://apps.who.int/iris/bitstream/handle/10665/259386/9789241550086-eng.pdf (accessed on 15 February 2025).
8. Sankar, M.J.; Sinha, B.; Chowdhury, R.; Bhandari, N.; Taneja, S.; Martines, J.; Bahl, R. Optimal breastfeeding practices and infant and child mortality: A systematic review and meta-analysis. *Acta Paediatr.* **2015**, *104*, 3–13. [CrossRef]
9. Yan, J.; Liu, L.; Zhu, Y.; Huang, G.; Wang, P.P. The association between breastfeeding and childhood obesity: A meta-analysis. *BMC Public Health* **2014**, *14*, 1267. [CrossRef]
10. Weng, S.F.; A Redsell, S.; A Swift, J.; Yang, M.; Glazebrook, C.P. Systematic review and meta-analyses of risk factors for childhood overweight identifiable during infancy. *Arch. Dis. Child.* **2012**, *97*, 1019–1026. [CrossRef]
11. Ip, S.; Chung, M.; Raman, G.; Trikalinos, T.A.; Lau, J. A summary of the Agency for Healthcare Research and Quality's evidence report on breastfeeding in developed countries. *Breastfeed. Med.* **2009**, *4* (Suppl. S1), S17. [CrossRef]
12. Hylander, M.A.; Strobino, D.M.; Dhanireddy, R. Human Milk Feedings and Infection Among Very Low Birth Weight Infants. *Pediatrics* **1998**, *102*, e38. [CrossRef] [PubMed]
13. Schanler, R.J. The use of human milk for premature infants. *Pediatr. Clin. N. Am.* **2001**, *48*, 207–219. [CrossRef]
14. Okamoto, T.; Shirai, M.; Kokubo, M.; Takahashi, S.; Kajino, M.; Takase, M.; Sakata, H.; Oki, J. Human milk reduces the risk of retinal detachment in extremely low-birthweight infants. *Pediatr. Int.* **2007**, *49*, 894–897. [CrossRef] [PubMed]
15. Vohr, B.R.; Poindexter, B.B.; Dusick, A.M.; McKinley, L.T.; Wright, L.L.; Langer, J.C.; Poole, W.K.; NICHD Neonatal Research Network. Beneficial effects of breast milk in the neonatal intensive care unit on the developmental outcome of extremely low birth weight infants at 18 months of age. *Pediatrics* **2006**, *118*, e115–e123. [CrossRef]
16. O'Connor, D.L.; Jacobs, J.; Hall, R.; Adamkin, D.; Auestad, N.; Castillo, M.; Connor, W.E.; Connor, S.L.; Fitzgerald, K.; Groh-Wargo, S.; et al. Growth and development of premature infants fed predominantly human milk, predominantly premature infant formula, or a combination of human milk and premature formula. *J. Pediatr. Gastroenterol. Nutr.* **2003**, *37*, 437–446. [CrossRef]
17. El-Khuffash, A.; Lewandowski, A.J.; Jain, A.; Hamvas, A.; Singh, G.K.; Levy, P.T. Cardiac Performance in the First Year of Age Among Preterm Infants Fed Maternal Breast Milk. *JAMA Netw. Open* **2021**, *4*, e2121206. [CrossRef] [PubMed]
18. Hart, A.; Lentine, K.L.; Smith, J.M.; Miller, J.M.; Skeans, M.A.; Prentice, M.; Robinson, A.; Foutz, J.; Booker, S.E.; Israni, A.K.; et al. OPTN/SRTR 2019 Annual Data Report: Kidney. *Am. J. Transplant.* **2021**, *21*, 21–137. [CrossRef]
19. Halloran, P.F. T Cell-mediated rejection of kidney transplants: A personal viewpoint. *Am. J. Transplant.* **2010**, *10*, 1126–1134. [CrossRef]
20. Loupy, A.; Lefaucheur, C. Antibody-Mediated Rejection of Solid-Organ Allografts. *N. Engl. J. Med.* **2018**, *379*, 1150–1160. [CrossRef]
21. Balani, S.S.; Jensen, C.J.; Kouri, A.M.; Kizilbash, S.J. Induction and maintenance immunosuppression in pediatric kidney transplantation—Advances and controversies. *Pediatr. Transplant.* **2021**, *25*, e14077. [CrossRef]
22. Parlakpinar, H.; Gunata, M. Transplantation and immunosuppression: A review of novel transplant-related immunosuppressant drugs. *Immunopharmacol. Immunotoxicol.* **2021**, *43*, 651–665. [CrossRef] [PubMed]
23. Chang, S.H.; Russ, G.R.; Chadban, S.J.; Campbell, S.B.; McDonald, S.P. Trends in kidney transplantation in Australia and New Zealand, 1993–2004. *Transplantation* **2007**, *84*, 611–618. [CrossRef]
24. Meier-Kriesche, H.-U.; Schold, J.D.; Kaplan, B. Long-term renal allograft survival: Have we made significant progress or is it time to rethink our analytic and therapeutic strategies? *Am. J. Transplant.* **2004**, *4*, 1289–1295. [CrossRef] [PubMed]
25. Halloran, P.F. Immunosuppressive Drugs for Kidney Transplantation. *N. Engl. J. Med.* **2004**, *351*, 2715–2729. [CrossRef]
26. Szumilas, K.; Wilk, A.; Wiśniewski, P.; Gimpel, A.; Dziedziejko, V.; Kipp, M.; Pawlik, A. Current Status Regarding Immunosuppressive Treatment in Patients after Renal Transplantation. *Int. J. Mol. Sci.* **2023**, *24*, 10301. [CrossRef]

27. Broen, J.C.A.; Van Laar, J.M. Mycophenolate mofetil, azathioprine and tacrolimus: Mechanisms in rheumatology. *Nat. Rev. Rheumatol.* **2020**, *16*, 167–178. [CrossRef] [PubMed]
28. Rhen, T.; Cidlowski, J.A. Antiinflammatory Action of Glucocorticoids—New Mechanisms for Old Drugs. *N. Engl. J. Med.* **2005**, *353*, 1711–1723. [CrossRef]
29. McKay, D.B.; Josephson, M.A. Reproduction and Transplantation: Report on the AST Consensus Conference on Reproductive Issues and Transplantation. *Am. J. Transplant.* **2005**, *5*, 1592–1599. [CrossRef]
30. Klein, C.L.; Josephson, M.A. Post-Transplant Pregnancy and Contraception. *Clin. J. Am. Soc. Nephrol.* **2022**, *17*, 114–120. [CrossRef]
31. Ponticelli, C.; Zaina, B.; Moroni, G. Planned Pregnancy in Kidney Transplantation. A Calculated Risk. *J. Pers. Med.* **2021**, *11*, 956. [CrossRef]
32. Shah, S.; Venkatesan, R.L.; Gupta, A.; Sanghavi, M.K.; Welge, J.; Johansen, R.; Kean, E.B.; Kaur, T.; Gupta, A.; Grant, T.J.; et al. Pregnancy outcomes in women with kidney transplant: Metaanalysis and systematic review. *BMC Nephrol.* **2019**, *20*, 24. [CrossRef] [PubMed]
33. Shah, S.; Verma, P. Overview of Pregnancy in Renal Transplant Patients. *Int. J. Nephrol.* **2016**, *2016*, 4539342. [CrossRef]
34. Newton, E.R.; Hale, T.W. Drugs in breast milk. *Clin. Obstet. Gynecol.* **2015**, *58*, 868–884. [CrossRef]
35. Drugs and Lactation Database (LactMed). Available online: https://www.ncbi.nlm.nih.gov/books/NBK547442/ (accessed on 3 March 2025).
36. Ziegenhagen, D.J.; Crombach, G.; Dieckmann, M.; Zehnter, E.; Wienand, P.; Baldamus, C.A. Pregnancy during cyclosporin medication following a kidney transplant. *Dtsch Med. Wochenschr.* **1988**, *113*, 260–263. [CrossRef]
37. Xu, L.-G.; Han, S.; Liu, Y.; Wang, H.-W.; Yang, Y.-R.; Qiu, F.; Peng, W.-L.; Tang, L.-G. Timing, conditions, and complications of post-operative conception and pregnancy in female renal transplant recipients. *Cell Biochem. Biophys.* **2011**, *61*, 421–426. [CrossRef] [PubMed]
38. Di Loreto, P.; Martino, F.; Chiaramonte, S.; Dissegna, D.; Ronco, C.; Marchesoni, D.; Catapano, P.; Romano, G.; Montanaro, D. Pregnancy after kidney transplantation: Two transplantation centers—Vicenza–udine experience. *Transplant. Proc.* **2010**, *42*, 1158–1161. [CrossRef]
39. Thomson, A.W.; Bonham, C.A.; Zeevi, A. Mode of action of tacrolimus (FK506): Molecular and cellular mechanisms. *Ther. Drug Monit.* **1995**, *17*, 584–591. [CrossRef]
40. Shah, S.; Ginat, D.T. Calcineurin Inhibitors. In *Neuroimaging Pharmacopoeia*, 2nd ed.; Springer: Cham, Switzerland, 2023; pp. 173–183. [CrossRef]
41. Gow, P.J.; Ghabrial, H.; Smallwood, R.A.; Morgan, D.J.; Ching, M.S. Neonatal hepatic drug elimination. *Pharmacol. Toxicol.* **2001**, *88*, 3–15. [CrossRef] [PubMed]
42. Cyclosporine. Drugs and Lactation Database (LactMed®). September 2024. Available online: https://www.ncbi.nlm.nih.gov/books/NBK501683/ (accessed on 14 February 2025).
43. van der Woude, C.; Ardizzone, S.; Bengtson, M.; Fiorino, G.; Fraser, G.; Katsanos, K.; Kolacek, S.; Juillerat, P.; Mulders, A.; Pedersen, N.; et al. The Second European Evidenced-Based Consensus on Reproduction and Pregnancy in Inflammatory Bowel Disease. *J. Crohn's Colitis* **2015**, *9*, 107–124. [CrossRef]
44. Thiagarajan, K.-F.; Arakali, S.R.; Mealey, K.J.; Cardonick, E.H.; Gaughan, W.J.; Davison, J.M.; Moritz, M.J.; Armenti, V.T. Safety considerations: Breastfeeding after transplant. *Prog. Transplant.* **2013**, *23*, 137–146. [CrossRef]
45. Türkmen, M.A.; Kavukçu, S.; Sarıoğlu, S.; Soylu, A.; Akhunlar, H.; Yılmaz, O.; Güven, H. Effects of lactational cyclosporine A use on rat pups. *Pediatr. Transplant.* **2006**, *10*, 454–460. [CrossRef] [PubMed]
46. Zaza, G.; Cheok, M.; Krynetskaia, N.; Thorn, C.; Stocco, G.; Hebert, J.M.; McLeod, H.; Weinshilboum, R.M.; Relling, M.V.; Evans, W.E.; et al. Thiopurine pathway. *Pharmacogenet. Genom.* **2010**, *20*, 573–574. [CrossRef]
47. Van Os, E.C.; Zins, B.J.; Sandborn, W.J.; Mays, D.C.; Tremaine, W.J.; Mahoney, D.W.; Zinsmeister, A.R.; Lipsky, J.J. Azathioprine pharmacokinetics after intravenous, oral, delayed release oral and rectal foam administration. *Gut* **1996**, *39*, 63–68. [CrossRef] [PubMed]
48. Chaudhary, D.; Jhaj, R. A case report on azathioprine-induced euprolactinemic galactorrhea. *Indian J. Pharmacol.* **2021**, *53*, 234–235. [CrossRef]
49. Uygur-Bayramiçli, O.; Aydin, D.; Ak, Ö.; Karadayi, N. Hyperprolactinemia caused by azathioprine. *J. Clin. Gastroenterol.* **2003**, *36*, 79–80. [CrossRef]
50. Nielsen, O.H.; Maxwell, C.; Hendel, J. IBD medications during pregnancy and lactation. *Nat. Rev. Gastroenterol. Hepatol.* **2014**, *11*, 116–127. [CrossRef]
51. Constantinescu, S.; Pai, A.; Coscia, L.A.; Davison, J.M.; Moritz, M.J.; Armenti, V.T. Breast-feeding after transplantation. *Best Pr. Res. Clin. Obstet. Gynaecol.* **2014**, *28*, 1163–1173. [CrossRef]
52. Flint, J.; Panchal, S.; Hurrell, A.; van de Venne, M.; Gayed, M.; Schreiber, K.; Arthanari, S.; Cunningham, J.; Flanders, L.; Moore, L.; et al. BSR and BHPR guideline on prescribing drugs in pregnancy and breastfeeding—Part I: Standard and biologic disease modifying anti-rheumatic drugs and corticosteroids. *Rheumatology* **2016**, *55*, 1693–1697. [CrossRef]

53. Lewis, G.J.; A Lamont, C.; A Lee, H.; Slapak, M. Successful pregnancy in a renal transplant recipient taking cyclosporin A. *BMJ* **1983**, *286*, 603. [CrossRef]
54. Flechner, S.M.; Katz, A.R.; Rogers, A.; Van Buren, C.; Kahan, B.D. The presence of cyclosporine in body tissues and fluids during pregnancy. *Am. J. Kidney Dis.* **1985**, *5*, 60–63. [CrossRef]
55. Moretti, M.; Ito, S.; Koren, G. Therapeutic drug monitoring in the lactating patient. *Reprod. Toxicol.* **1995**, *9*, 580–581. [CrossRef]
56. Thiru, Y.; Bateman, D.N.; Coulthard, M.G. Drug points: Successful breast feeding while mother was taking cyclosporin. *BMJ* **1997**, *315*, 463. [CrossRef]
57. Nyberg, G.; Haljamäe, U.; Frisenette-Fich, C.; Wennergren, M.; Kjellmer, I. Breast-feeding during treatment with cyclosporine. *Transplantation* **1998**, *65*, 253–255. [CrossRef] [PubMed]
58. Thiagarajan, K.D.; Easterling, T.; Davis, C.; Bond, E.F. Breast-feeding by a cyclosporine-treated mother. *Obstet. Gynecol.* **2001**, *97*, 816–818. [CrossRef]
59. Moretti, M.E.; Sgro, M.; Johnson, D.W.; Sauve, R.S.; Woolgar, M.J.; Taddio, A.; Verjee, Z.; Giesbrecht, E.; Koren, G.; Ito, S. Cyclosporine excretion into breast milk. *Transplantation* **2003**, *75*, 2144–2146. [CrossRef] [PubMed]
60. Osadchy, A.; Koren, G. Cyclosporine and lactation: When the mother is willing to breastfeed. *Ther. Drug Monit.* **2011**, *33*, 147–148. [CrossRef]
61. Adam, M. Cyclosporine and lactation. *Nephrology* **2011**, *16*, 249. [CrossRef]
62. Lahiff, C.; Moss, A.C. Cyclosporine in the management of severe ulcerative colitis while breast-feeding. *Inflamm. Bowel Dis.* **2011**, *17*, E78. [CrossRef]
63. Mazzuoccolo, L.D.; Andrada, R.; Pellerano, G.; Neglia, V.; Abeldaño, A. Levels of cyclosporine in breast milk and passage into the circulation of the infant of a mother with psoriasis. *Int. J. Dermatol.* **2014**, *53*, 355–356. [CrossRef]
64. Fiocchi, R.; D'elia, E.; Vittori, C.; Sebastiani, R.; Strobelt, N.; Eleftheriou, G.; Introna, M.; Freddi, C.; Crippa, A. First Report of a Successful Pregnancy in an Everolimus-Treated Heart-Transplanted Patient: Neonatal Disappearance of Immunosuppressive Drugs. *Am. J. Transplant.* **2016**, *16*, 1319–1322. [CrossRef]
65. Kociszewska-Najman, B.; Mazanowska, N.; Borek-Dzięcioł, B.; Pączek, L.; Samborowska, E.; Szpotańska-Sikorska, M.; Pietrzak, B.; Dadlez, M.; Wielgoś, M. Low Content of Cyclosporine A and Its Metabolites in the Colostrum of Post-Transplant Mothers. *Nutrients* **2020**, *12*, 2713. [CrossRef] [PubMed]
66. Li, R.; Zhang, C.; Wang, H.; An, Y. Breastfeeding by a mother taking cyclosporine for nephrotic syndrome. *Int. Breastfeed. J.* **2022**, *17*, 72. [CrossRef] [PubMed]
67. E French, A.; Soldin, S.J.; Soldin, O.P.; Koren, G. Milk Transfer and Neonatal Safety of Tacrolimus. *Ann. Pharmacother.* **2003**, *37*, 815–818. [CrossRef]
68. Gardiner, S.J.; Begg, E.J. Breastfeeding during tacrolimus therapy. *Obstet. Gynecol.* **2006**, *107 Pt 2*, 453–455. [CrossRef]
69. Jain, A.; Venkataramanan, R.; Fung, J.J.; Gartner, J.C.; Lever, J.; Balan, V.; Warty, V.; Starzl, T.E. Pregnancy after liver transplantation under tacrolimus. *Transplantation* **1997**, *64*, 559–565. [CrossRef]
70. Gouraud, A.; Bernard, N.; Millaret, A.; Bruel, M.; Paret, N.; Descotes, J.; Vial, T. Follow-up of tacrolimus breastfed babies. *Transplantation* **2012**, *94*, e38–e40. [CrossRef]
71. Gomez-Lobo, V.; Landy, H.J.; Matsumoto, C.; Fishbein, T.M. Pregnancy in an intestinal transplant recipient. *Obstet. Gynecol.* **2012**, *120*, 497–500. [CrossRef] [PubMed]
72. Bramham, K.; Chusney, G.; Lee, J.; Lightstone, L.; Nelson-Piercy, C. Breastfeeding and tacrolimus: Serial monitoring in breast-fed and bottle-fed infants. *Clin. J. Am. Soc. Nephrol.* **2013**, *8*, 563–567. [CrossRef]
73. Zheng, S.; Easterling, T.R.; Hays, K.; Umans, J.G.; Miodovnik, M.; Clark, S.; Calamia, J.C.; Thummel, K.E.; Shen, D.D.; Davis, C.L.; et al. Tacrolimus placental transfer at delivery and neonatal exposure through breast milk. *Br. J. Clin. Pharmacol.* **2013**, *76*, 988–996. [CrossRef]
74. Kociszewska-Najman, B.; Mazanowska, N.; Pietrzak, B.; Paczek, L.; Szpotanska-Sikorska, M.; Schreiber-Zamora, J.; Hryniewiecka, E.; Zochowska, D.; Samborowska, E.; Dadlez, M.; et al. Low Transfer of Tacrolimus and Its Metabolites into Colostrum of Graft Recipient Mothers. *Nutrients* **2018**, *10*, 267. [CrossRef]
75. Izumi, Y.; Miyashita, T.; Migita, K. Safety of Tacrolimus Treatment during Pregnancy and Lactation in Systemic Lupus Erythematosus: A Report of Two Patients. *Tohoku J. Exp. Med.* **2014**, *234*, 51–56. [CrossRef] [PubMed]
76. Hiramatsu, Y.; Yoshida, S.; Kotani, T.; Nakamura, E.; Kimura, Y.; Fujita, D.; Nagayasu, Y.; Shabana, K.; Makino, S.; Takeuchi, T.; et al. Changes in the blood level, efficacy, and safety of tacrolimus in pregnancy and the lactation period in patients with systemic lupus erythematosus. *Lupus* **2018**, *27*, 2245–2252. [CrossRef]
77. Akamine, Y.; Fujiyama, N.; Kagaya, H.; Saito, M.; Miura, H.; Terada, Y.; Takahashi, T.; Satoh, S.; Miura, M. Tacrolimus concentrations after renal transplantation in a mother-neonate dyad: Maternal, neonatal and breast milk measurements. *J. Clin. Pharm. Ther.* **2021**, *46*, 1800–1803. [CrossRef]
78. Kuczaj, A.; Danel, A.; Warwas, S.; Przybyłowski, P.; Śliwka, J.; Pawlak, S.; Trzcińska, I.; Hrapkowicz, T. Toxic Milk- Should We Still be Afraid of Breastfeeding While on Tacrolimus Therapy: A Case Study. *J. Heart Lung Transplant.* **2024**, *43*, S631. [CrossRef]

79. Kociszewska-Najman, B.; Szpotańska-Sikorska, M.; Mazanowska, N.; Pączek, L.; Samborowska, E.; Dadlez, M.; Wielgoś, M.; Pietrzak, B. Transfer of Everolimus into Colostrum of a Kidney Transplant Mother. *Ann. Transplant.* **2017**, *22*, 755–758. [CrossRef]
80. Coulam, C.B.; Moyer, T.P.; Jiang, N.S.; Zincke, H. Breast-feeding after renal transplantation. *Transpl. Proc.* **1982**, *14*, 605–609.
81. Grekas, D.M.; Vasiliou, S.S.; Lazarides, A.N. Immunosuppressive therapy and breast-feeding after renal transplantation. *Nephron* **1984**, *37*, 68. [CrossRef]
82. Gardiner, S.J.; Gearry, R.B.; Roberts, R.L.; Zhang, M.; Barclay, M.L.; Begg, E.J. Exposure to thiopurine drugs through breast milk is low based on metabolite concentrations in mother-infant pairs. *Br. J. Clin. Pharmacol.* **2006**, *62*, 453–456. [CrossRef] [PubMed]
83. E Moretti, M.; Verjee, Z.; Ito, S.; Koren, G. Breast-feeding during maternal use of azathioprine. *Ann. Pharmacother.* **2006**, *40*, 2269–2272. [CrossRef]
84. Sau, A.; Clarke, S.; Bass, J.; Kaiser, A.; Marinaki, A.; Nelson-Piercy, C. Azathioprine and breastfeeding—Is it safe? *BJOG* **2007**, *114*, 498–501. [CrossRef]
85. Christensen, L.A.; Dahlerup, J.F.; Nielsen, M.J.; Fallingborg, J.F.; Schmiegelow, K. Azathioprine treatment during lactation. *Aliment. Pharmacol. Ther.* **2008**, *28*, 1209–1213. [CrossRef] [PubMed]
86. Zelinkova, Z.; De Boer, I.P.; Van Dijke, M.J.; Kuipers, E.J.; Van Der Woude, C.J. Azathioprine treatment during lactation. *Aliment. Pharmacol. Ther.* **2009**, *30*, 90–91. [CrossRef]
87. Angelberger, S.; Reinisch, W.; Messerschmidt, A.; Miehsler, W.; Novacek, G.; Vogelsang, H.; Dejaco, C. Long-term follow-up of babies exposed to azathioprine in utero and via breastfeeding. *J. Crohn's Colitis* **2011**, *5*, 95–100. [CrossRef]
88. de Meij, T.G.J.; Jharap, B.; Kneepkens, C.M.F.; van Bodegraven, A.A.; de Boer, N.K.H.; Dutch Initiative on Crohn and Colitis. Long-term follow-up of children exposed intrauterine to maternal thiopurine therapy during pregnancy in females with inflammatory bowel disease. *Aliment. Pharmacol. Ther.* **2013**, *38*, 38–43. [CrossRef] [PubMed]
89. Katz, F.H.; Duncan, B.R. Entry of Prednisone into Human Milk. *N. Engl. J. Med.* **1975**, *293*, 1154. [CrossRef] [PubMed]
90. Sagraves, R.; Kaiser, D.; Sharpe, G.L. Prednisone and prednisolone concentrations in the milk of a lactating mother. *Drug Intell Clin. Pharm.* **1981**, *15*, 484. Available online: https://archive.org/details/sim_annals-of-pharmacotherapy_1981_15_index/mode/2up (accessed on 20 February 2025).
91. Öst, L.; Wettrell, G.; Björkhem, I.; Rane, A. Prednisolone excretion in human milk. *J. Pediatr.* **1985**, *106*, 1008–1011. [CrossRef]
92. A Greenberger, P.; Odeh, Y.K.; Frederiksen, M.C.; Atkinson, A.J. Pharmacokinetics of prednisolone transfer to breast milk. *Clin. Pharmacol. Ther.* **1993**, *53*, 324–328. [CrossRef]
93. Ryu, R.J.; Easterling, T.R.; Caritis, S.N.; Venkataramanan, R.; Umans, J.G.; Ahmed, M.S.; Clark, S.; Kantrowitz-Gordon, I.; Hays, K.; Bs, B.B.; et al. Prednisone Pharmacokinetics During Pregnancy and Lactation. *J. Clin. Pharmacol.* **2018**, *58*, 1223–1232. [CrossRef]
94. Klintmalm, G.B.; Gunby, R.T. Successful Pregnancy in a Liver Transplant Recipient on Belatacept. *Liver Transplant.* **2020**, *26*, 1193–1194. [CrossRef]
95. Coscia, L.R.; Cohen, D.; Dube, G.K.; Hofmann, R.M.; Moritz, M.J.; Gattis, S.P.D.; Basu, A.M. Outcomes With Belatacept Exposure During Pregnancy in Kidney Transplant Recipients: A Case Series. *Transplantation* **2023**, *107*, 2047–2054. [CrossRef]
96. Cuadrado-Payán, E.; Diekmann, F.; Cucchiari, D. Medical Aspects of mTOR Inhibition in Kidney Transplantation. *Int. J. Mol. Sci.* **2022**, *23*, 7707. [CrossRef]
97. McKinzie, C.J.; Casale, J.P.; Guerci, J.C.; Prom, A.; Doligalski, C.T. Outcomes of Children with Fetal and Lactation Immunosuppression Exposure Born to Female Transplant Recipients. *Pediatr. Drugs* **2022**, *24*, 483–497. [CrossRef]
98. Prednisone. Drugs and Lactation Database (LactMed®). April 2024. Available online: https://www.ncbi.nlm.nih.gov/books/NBK501077/ (accessed on 15 February 2025).
99. Hossen, M.; Ma, Y.; Yin, Z.; Xia, Y.; Du, J.; Huang, J.Y.; Huang, J.J.; Zou, L.; Ye, Z.; Huang, Z. Current understanding of CTLA-4: From mechanism to autoimmune diseases. *Front. Immunol.* **2023**, *14*, 1198365. [CrossRef]
100. Archdeacon, P.; Dixon, C.; Belen, O.; Albrecht, R.; Meyer, J. Summary of the US FDA approval of belatacept. *Am. J. Transplant.* **2012**, *12*, 554–562. [CrossRef] [PubMed]
101. European Medicines Agency (EMA). Available online: https://www.ema.europa.eu/en/medicines/human/EPAR/nulojix (accessed on 2 March 2025).
102. El Hennawy, H.M.; Safar, O.; Al Faifi, A.S.; El Nazer, W.; Kamal, A.; Mahedy, A.; Zaitoun, M.; Fahmy, A.E.; Wageh, A. Belatacept rescue therapy of CNI-induced nephrotoxicity, meta-analysis. *Transplant. Rev.* **2021**, *35*, 100653. [CrossRef]
103. Cockfield, S.M.; Wilson, S.; Campbell, P.M.; Cantarovich, M.; Gangji, A.; Houde, I.; Jevnikar, A.M.; Keough-Ryan, T.M.; Monroy-Cuadros, F.-M.; Nickerson, P.W.; et al. Comparison of the effects of standard vs low-dose prolonged-release tacrolimus with or without ACEi/ARB on the histology and function of renal allografts. *Am. J. Transplant.* **2019**, *19*, 1730–1744. [CrossRef]
104. Rodriguez-Ramirez, S.; Al Jurdi, A.; Konvalinka, A.; Riella, L.V. Antibody-mediated rejection: Prevention, monitoring and treatment dilemmas. *Curr. Opin. Organ Transplant.* **2022**, *27*, 405–414. [CrossRef]

105. Wind, M.; Gaasbeek, A.; Oosten, L.; Rabelink, T.; van Lith, J.; Sueters, M.; Teng, Y. Therapeutic plasma exchange in pregnancy: A literature review. *Eur. J. Obstet. Gynecol. Reprod. Biol.* **2021**, *260*, 29–36. [CrossRef]
106. Agarwal, K.A.; Pavlakis, M. Sexuality, Contraception, and Pregnancy in Kidney Transplantation. *Kidney Med.* **2021**, *3*, 837–847. [CrossRef]

Journal of
Clinical Medicine

MDPI

Article

Exploring Net Immunosuppressive Status with Torque Teno Virus Viral Load in Kidney Transplant Recipients with High Molecular Injury

Emilio Rodrigo [1,*], Elena González-López [2], Javier Gonzalo Ocejo-Vinyals [2], Enrique Pasache [1], Cristina García-Majado [1], Covadonga López del Moral [1], Ana García-Santiago [1], Adalberto Benito-Hernández [1], María Victoria Francia [3] and Juan Carlos Ruiz [1]

1 Immunopathology Group, Nephrology Department, Marqués de Valdecilla University Hospital-IDIVAL, University of Cantabria, 39005 Santander, Spain; juancarlos.ruiz@scsalud.es (J.C.R.)
2 Immunopathology Group, Immunology Department, Marqués de Valdecilla University Hospital-IDIVAL, University of Cantabria, 39005 Santander, Spain; egonzalezlope@saludcastillayleon.es (E.G.-L.); javiergonzalo.ocejo@scsalud.es (J.G.O.-V.)
3 Infectious Diseases and Clinical Microbiology Group, Marqués de Valdecilla University Hospital-IDIVAL, University of Cantabria, 39005 Santander, Spain
* Correspondence: emilio.rodrigo@scsalud.es; Tel.: +34-942202738

Abstract: Background/Objectives: New monitoring methods are being developed to improve the kidney transplant outcome. Among them, the measurement of Torque Teno virus load (TTV load) has been associated with the overall immunosuppressive status and the percentage of donor-derived circulating free DNA (dd-cfDNA) with molecular graft injury, mainly related to antibody-mediated rejection (AbMR). Both methods provide complementary information, but they have not been previously used together for the monitoring of kidney transplant recipients (KTx). **Methods**: A prospective study including 42 KTx performed in our centre was conducted, in which we monitored dd-cfDNA using a targeted NGS assay (AlloSeq cfDNA) in the first month and the TTV load with in-house PCR in the first and third months. **Results**: Eleven KTx with high molecular injury defined by dd-cfDNA $\geq$ 1.0% were selected. The TTV load showed a non-significant trend of being lower in AbMR patients (2.91, IQR 4.18 vs. 3.48, IQR 1.47 log10 copies/mL, $p = 0.788$). No overimmunosuppressed patient developed AbMR, whereas 40% of non-overimmunosuppressed patients showed AbMR ($p = 0.428$). The TTV load increased more in the AbMR-treated KTx (0.00, IQR 4.71 vs. +6.58, IQR 4.04 log10 copies/mL, $p = 0.042$) from months one to three, with all AbMR-treated KTx becoming overimmunosuppressed. KTx with opportunistic infections showed higher TTV loads in the third month (5.18, IQR 5.92 vs. 11.53, IQR 3.54 log10 copies/mL, $p = 0.024$). **Conclusions**: KTx with molecular injury secondary to rejection tended to be less immunosuppressed, as indicated by a low TTV load. After AbMR therapy, all KTx became overimmunosuppressed and suffered a higher risk of opportunistic infections. Dual monitoring provides useful complementary information for the follow-up of kidney transplant recipients.

Keywords: antibody-mediated rejection; donor-derived cell-free DNA; immune response; infection; kidney transplantation; monitoring; Torque Teno virus

1. Introduction

In the monitoring of kidney transplant recipients, physicians attempt to hold patients at an optimal level of immunosuppression to avoid both the risks associated with overimmunosuppression, mainly infections and cancer, and the risk of triggering an alloimmune response and subsequent rejection if the level of immunosuppression is low [1–3]. Along with monitoring certain levels through laboratory tests, such as renal function and albuminuria, and tracking the appearances and titres of newly introduced donor-specific antibodies, the usual practice is to monitor trough blood levels of calcineurin-lowering drugs, attempting to hold them within a narrow therapeutic range. However, it is known that the levels of calcineurin inhibitors are more related to the risk of presenting side effects than the risk of rejection [4]. Some centres perform follow-up biopsies to better identify the status of the renal graft, but this is an invasive technique with potential risks [5]. Hence, it is of great interest to develop new non-invasive monitoring tools that will allow for improved knowledge about the immunological statuses of kidney transplant patients.

In recent years, two new methods of monitoring solid organ transplants have been developed. First, the net immunosuppressive state can be estimated by measuring Torque Teno virus (TTV) levels in the blood. TTV is a member of the Anelloviridae family, which is ubiquitous and non-pathogenic to humans [6]. High TTV loads are associated with a higher risk of infection and other immunosuppressive side effects, whereas low TTV loads are associated with a higher risk of acute rejection in kidney and other solid organ transplants [7,8]. The Vienna group proposed using cut-off values <4.6 log10 c/mL and >6.6 log10 copies/mL to identify kidney transplant recipients with under- and overimmunosuppressive statuses [6]. Elsewhere, the percentage of donor-derived cell-free DNA (dd-cfDNA) has been proposed as a potential biomarker of acute rejection and graft failure in kidney transplantation [9]. Elevated dd-cfDNA levels have been associated with an increased risk of renal graft damage, specifically polyomavirus nephropathy, acute cellular rejection, and, primarily, antibody-mediated rejection (AbMR) [10–13]. A percentage of dd-cfDNA above 1% is highly suggestive of AbMR, allowing the identification of the group of patients with high molecular damage of the graft [14]. In a previous study, we used dd-cfDNA measurement to identify kidney transplant recipients with greater molecular damage and, therefore, a higher risk of rejection or infection in the kidney graft [12]. The aim of the present study was to analyse whether the simultaneous measurement of the TTV viral load allows us to differentiate which of these patients had underimmunosuppression (acute rejection risk) or overimmunosuppression (infection risk) in order to identify the causes of the molecular graft injury in a non-invasive manner.

2. Materials and Methods

We conducted a prospective study including the kidney transplants performed in University Hospital Marqués de Valdecilla from January 2021 to April 2022. All participants were adults and gave written informed consent before undergoing kidney transplantation, which was performed in accordance with the tenets of the Declaration of Helsinki and with the approval of the Regional Ethics Committee of our institution (reference number: PI20/01710). Patients who had received non-kidney solid organ transplants, those from uncontrolled cardiac death donations or from living donors, those with pre-formed donor-specific antibodies, and those with a panel-reactive antibody level greater than 98% were excluded.

Relevant information on the characteristics of the recipient, the donor, and the graft was collected. All acute rejection episodes were confirmed by biopsy. Indicative biopsies were performed if the creatinine level increased by 25% or more from the previous value or if proteinuria persisted at >1 g per day. We considered opportunistic infections to be those associated with cellular and humoral immunosuppression, including viral (CMV, EBV, HSV, VZV, BK polyomavirus-associated nephropathy and recurrent hepatitis, HBV, HCV), bacterial (typical and atypical mycobacteria, others such as Nocardia, Listeria, etc.), and fungal (Pneumocystis jirovecii pneumonia, Candida, and invasive fungal infections) infections. The detection of viral, bacterial, and fungal infections was accomplished through the utilisation of standard microbiological techniques.

Maintenance immunosuppressive therapy consisted of twice-daily tacrolimus, mycophenolate mofetil, and prednisone. Recipients at risk of delayed graft function or/and receiving a graft from an expanded criteria donor were treated with Basiliximab. Kidney transplant recipients with a higher rejection risk due to hypersensitisation or previous graft loss due to acute rejection received induction with thymoglobulin. All patients were administered trimethoprim-sulfamethoxazole for six months as prophylaxis against Pneumocystis jirovecii pneumonia. Valganciclovir was used for three months in CMV IgG-negative recipients of a CMV IgG-positive donor and in those patients who received induction with thymoglobulin.

Plasma tacrolimus concentrations (μg/L) were measured by chemiluminescent microparticle immunoassay using the Architect iSystem (CMIA; Abbott Laboratories, Abbott Park, IL, USA). Trough tacrolimus blood concentrations were adjusted to be between 8 and 12 ng/mL until the third month. Trough mycophenolic acid (MPA) concentrations (mg/L) were quantified by homogeneous enzyme-linked immunosorbent assay (Emit 2000 Mycophenolic Acid Assay; Siemens, Munich, Germany) at month 1. Samples for TTV load measurement were obtained before transplantation and at days 30 and 90 post-transplantation. TTV viral load was determined in duplicate using a recently validated protocol with the commercial TTV R-GENE® kit (bioMérieux, Craponne, France), as previously reported [15,16]. Under- and overimmunosuppressive statuses were defined according to a TTV viral load <4.6 log10 c/mL or above 6.6 log10 copies/mL [6].

Peripheral blood samples were collected in Streck Cell-Free DNA BCT tubes one month after the transplant, in order to determine the relative amount of circulating donor-derived cell-free DNA (dd-cfDNA). This was achieved using a targeted NGS assay that utilised 202 single nucleotide polymorphisms (AlloSeq cfDNA, CareDx, Inc., Brisbane, CA, USA) [12]. According to the manufacturer's instructions, a cut-off of 1.0% was used as an abnormal dd-cfDNA result to define "high molecular injury" [14]. We included 42 patients in this study for whom dd-cfDNA levels and TTV viral loads were available at one-month post-transplant.

To express continuous variables, the median and interquartile range (IQR) were utilised; relative frequencies were employed to characterise categorical variables. The Mann–Whitney U test was used to compare continuous variables between dichotomous data, and the chi-squared test was used to examine the relationship between two qualitative variables. Paired TTV loads were compared using the Wilcoxon signed rank test. Univariate and multivariate regression analyses were performed to assess the variables associated with TTV load in the third month and the differences in TTV load between months 1 and 3. A p-value less than 0.05 was considered statistically significant. Statistical analyses were performed with SPSS version 22.0 (SPSS, Inc., Chicago, IL, USA).

3. Results

Among 42 kidney transplant recipients with dd-cfDNA measured in the first month, we selected 11 with a high molecular injury defined by dd-cfDNA $\geq$ 1.0%. The main patient characteristics of these 11 patients and a comparison with the whole group are shown in Table 1. The results mentioned in the following paragraphs refer exclusively to these 11 selected patients. TTV load increased progressively from baseline (2.45, IQR 2.00–2.77 log10 copies/mL) to months 1 (3.20, IQR 2.09–5.42 log10 copies/mL, $p = 0.008$) and 3 (7.84, IQR 2.99–11.01 log10 copies/mL, $p = 0.037$) (Figure 1). There were one (9.1%) and six (54.5%) overimmunosuppressed patients in the first and third months, respectively.

Conversely, eight (72.7%) and three (27.3%) patients were underimmunosuppressed in the first and third months, respectively.

Table 1. Main patient characteristics.

Number of Patients	11	31	p
Recipient age (years)	60.0 [48.0–73.0]	59.0 [47.0–66.0]	0.572
Recipient sex (male)	63.6%	80.6%	0.255
Diabetic nephropathy	18.2%	25.8%	0.610
Time in renal replacement therapy (months)	24.5 [10.5–108.7]	10.7 [0.0–32.6]	0.062
Retransplant	36.4%	12.9%	0.089
Pre-emptive transplantation	18.2%	22.6%	0.760
Donor age (years)	61.0 [47.0–65.0]	58.0 [47.0–65.0]	0.910
Antigen HLA Class-I and -II mismatches	8.0 [7.0–9.0]	7.0 [5.0–9.0]	0.233
Cold ischaemia time (h)	20.0 [18.0–24.0]	22.0 [17.0–24.0]	0.822
Induction	72.7%	64.5%	0.620
Thymoglobulin (%)	45.5%	16.1%	0.050
Basiliximab (%)	27.3%	48.4%	0.224
Delayed graft function (%)	36.4%	22.6%	0.372
1-month AbMR	36.4%	3.2%	0.004
Infection from months 1 to 3	36.4%	41.9%	0.746
Opportunistic infection from months 1 to 3	27.3%	12.9%	0.272
First-month eGFR (mL/min/1.73 m^2)	43.0 [28.0–54.0]	51.0 [42.0–72.0]	0.138
1-year eGFR (mL/min/1.73 m^2)	45.0 [38.0–49.0]	50.0 [38.0–71.8]	0.514
First-month mean Tacrolimus trough level (ng/mL)	12.5 [11.4–14.3]	12.3 [11.2–14.2]	0.822
Tacrolimus trough level at month 1 (ng/mL)	13.0 [10.0–15.0]	12.0 [9.0–14.0]	0.233
Mycophenolic acid trough level at month 1 (ng/mL)	2.0 [1.8–4.0]	2.0 [1.0–3.0]	0.569
First-month TTV load (log10 copies/mL)	3.20 [2.09–5.41]	2.23 [1.18–3.28]	0.117
Third-month TTV load (log10 copies/mL)	7.84 [3.00–11.01]	5.72 [2.85–8.59]	0.295

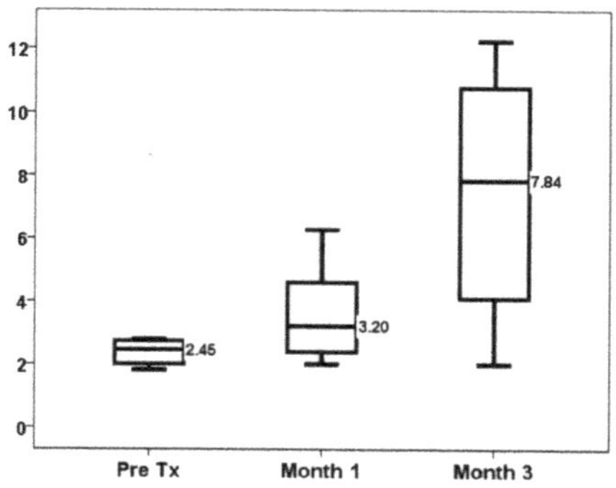

Figure 1. Kinetics of TTV load (log10 copies/mL).

There was no significant difference in TTV load at month one between patients receiving or not receiving induction therapy (2.95, IQR 2.98 log10 copies/mL vs. 3.77,

IQR 3.36 log10 copies/mL, $p = 0.376$). While the differences were also not significant at month three, there was a trend in patients receiving induction therapy of showing a higher TTV load (9.23, range 6.27 log10 copies/mL vs. 2.99, range 5.84 log10 copies/mL, $p = 0.133$). Only one patient (12.5%) receiving induction was overimmunosuppressed at month one, whereas none of the patients not receiving induction were overimmunosuppressed at month one ($p = 0.521$). At month three, five (62.5%) patients treated with induction became overimmunosuppressed, while one (33.3%) patient who did not receive induction was overimmunosuppressed ($p = 0.387$). Conversely, underimmunosuppression was observed in one (33.3%) and two (25.0%) recipients at month one ($p = 0.782$) and in seven (87.5%) and one (33.3%) recipients at month three ($p = 0.072$), respectively, with and without induction therapy.

Four patients suffered AbMR and four more patients suffered different complications that could justify the high molecular injury (three patients required procedures on the graft due to hydronephrosis, one of whom suffered graft pyelonephritis caused by Klebsiella sp, and another patient presented with cytomegalovirus infection in the first month post-transplant). TTV loads in the first month were not different between patients with and without antibody-mediated rejection (2.91, IQR 4.18 log10 copies/mL vs. 3.48, IQR 1.47 log10 copies/mL, $p = 0.788$). Although 50% of underimmunosuppressed patients and none of the patients without underimmunosuppression suffered AbMR, the differences were not statistically significant ($p = 0.125$). No overimmunosuppressed patients developed AbMR, while 40% of non-overimmunosuppressed patients showed AbMR ($p = 0.428$). The AbMR rate was comparable between patients who received induction therapy and those who did not (37.5% vs. 33.3%, $p = 0.898$).

From months one to three, four (36.4%) patients developed at least one infection episode, with three (27.3%) of them opportunistic infections. Similarly, there were no differences in the risk of suffering infection (2.91, IQR 3.42 log10 copies/mL vs. 3.77, IQR 6.53 log10 copies/mL, $p = 0.412$) before month three or opportunistic infection (3.06, IQR 3.88 log10 copies/mL vs. 3.76, IQR 1.68 log10 copies/mL, $p = 1.000$) according to the TTV load in the first month. Overimmunosuppressed patients did not suffer a statistically significantly higher number of infections (30% vs. 100%, $p = 0.165$) or opportunistic infections (40% vs. 0%, $p = 0.521$). The infection rates (37.5% vs. 33.3%, $p = 0.898$) and the rates of opportunistic infection from months one to three (25.0% vs. 33.3%, $p = 0.782$) were not found to be significantly different between patients receiving and not receiving induction therapy.

As previously reported, the TTV load increased up to month three. Four patients with AbMR received specific therapy with plasmapheresis and IVIg following the recommendations [17]. TTV load in the third month showed a trend of being higher in patients who received AbMR therapy (5.18, IQR 8.55 log10 copies/mL vs. 9.47, IQR 4.06 log10 copies/mL, $p = 0.109$) (Figure 2). The difference in TTV load between months one and three was significantly higher in the AbMR-treated kidney transplant recipients (0.00, IQR 4.71 log10 copies/mL vs. +6.58, IQR 4.04 log10 copies/mL, $p = 0.042$) (Figure 3). All treated patients became overimmunosuppressed, whereas the rate of overimmunosuppression was 28.6% in non-treated patients (0.022) (Figure 4). Univariate linear regression analysis revealed a correlation between AbMR therapy and increased TTV load variations between months one and three (β 0.642, 95%CI 0.529–10.005, $p = 0.033$). To determine whether this influence could be related to the induction therapy, we performed a multivariate analysis, which revealed that AbMR therapy was associated (β 0.624, 95%CI 1.120–9.110, $p = 0.01$) with a higher increase in TTV load between month one and three, independently of induction therapy (β 0.481, 95%CI −0.059–8.571, $p = 0.053$).

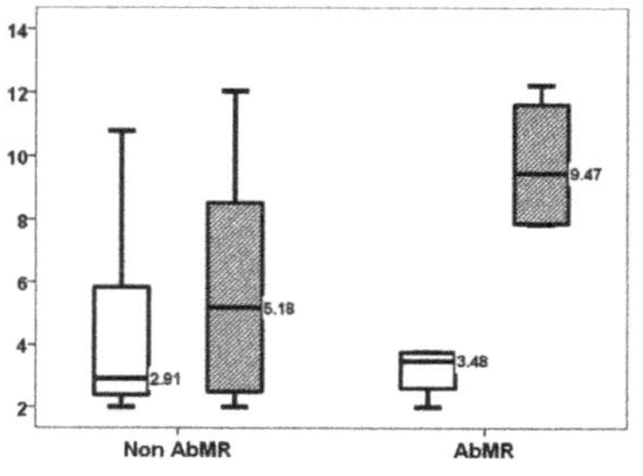

Figure 2. TTV load (log10 copies/mL) at 1st month (white bars) and 3rd month (stripped bars) in patients with and without AbMR.

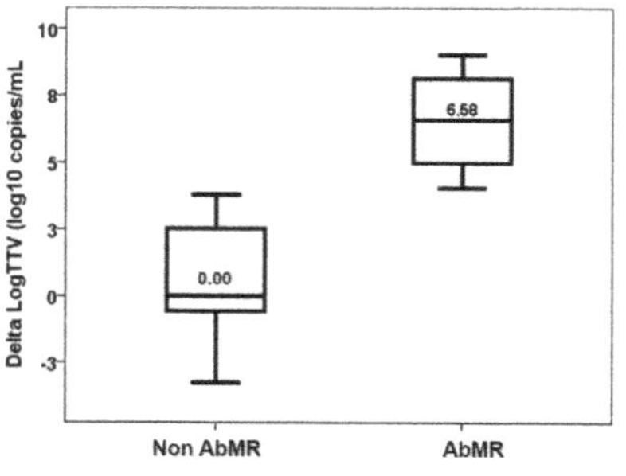

Figure 3. Delta LogTTV (log10 copies/mL) in patients with and without AbMR (p = 0.042).

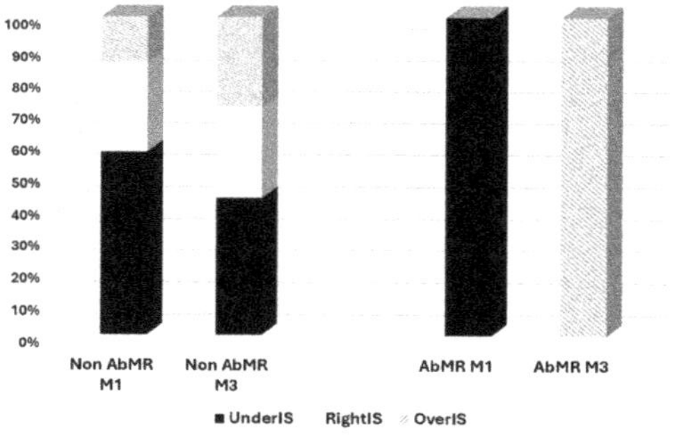

Figure 4. Classification according to the immunosuppressive level in patients receiving or not receiving AbMR therapy. Non AbMR = no diagnosis of antibody-mediated rejection; AbMR = antibody-mediated rejection; M1 = month 1; M3 = month 3; UnderIS = underimmunosuppressive status, OverIS = overimmunosuppressive status; RightIS = right immunosuppressive status.

Eight patients (72.7%) developed at least one infection episode and four developed opportunistic infections (36.4%) between months three and six. TTV load in the third month was not significantly different between patients without and with infection between months three and six (2.99, IQR 4.5 log10 copies/mL vs. 9.23, IQR 5.93 log10 copies/mL, p = 0.085). Those with opportunistic infections showed higher TTV loads in the third month (5.18, IQR 5.92 log10 copies/mL vs. 11.53, IQR 3.54 log10 copies/mL, p = 0.024) (Figure 5). Overimmunosuppressed patients suffered a significantly higher rate of infections (40.0% vs. 100.0%, p = 0.026) and opportunistic infections (0.0% vs. 66.7%, p = 0.022) between months three and six. The infection rates (87.5% vs. 33.3%, p = 0.072) and the rates of opportunistic infection between months three and six (37.5% vs. 33.3%, p = 0.898) were not significantly different in patients receiving induction therapy compared to those not receiving it. Univariate linear regression analysis showed that TTV load in the third month was higher in patients who developed opportunistic infections between the third and sixth months (β 3.021, 95%CI 1.374–9.574, $p = 0.014$). After multivariate analysis, kidney transplant recipients who developed opportunistic infections between months three and six showed higher TTV loads (β 3.726, 95%CI 2.033–8.635, $p = 0.006$) independently of induction therapy (β 2.539, 95%CI 0.360–7.491, $p = 0.035$).

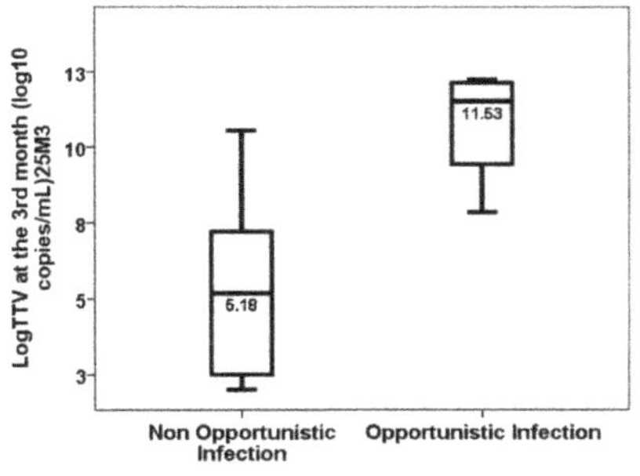

Figure 5. LogTTV (log10 copies/mL) in the 3rd month in patients with and without opportunistic infection between months 3 and 6.

4. Discussion

The development of new monitoring methods for solid organ transplants can facilitate their follow-up and improve long-term outcomes by allowing earlier and minimally invasive detection of both rejection and infection risk. Many of these new markers offer complementary information, and their combined use could be of great help in addition to conventional monitoring [18]. For example, a higher percentage of donor-derived cell-free DNA circulating in the recipient's blood has been associated with a higher risk of current or future rejection, especially AbMR. It can also be used as a marker of response to rejection treatment and of the risk of infections in the renal graft [9–14,19–22]. On the other hand, the measurement of TTV viral load allows the global state of immunosuppression of the patient to be assessed and thus the identification of whether they are at risk of developing rejection if they are underimmunosuppressed, or infection if they are overimmunosuppressed [6–8]. In this regard, we carried out for the first time a dual monitoring using dd-cfDNA and TTV viral load in kidney transplant recipients with the aim of identifying which patients were experiencing molecular damage in the kidney graft and differentiating whether the cause of the damage was infectious or secondary to the alloimmune response, based on the estimated global level of immunosuppression using the TTV viral load. Interestingly, we found that patients with high molecular damage who were experiencing rejection tended to have lower TTV viral load levels, although the small number of patients studied limited the degree to which the results could reach statistical significance. Similarly, only patients with low TTV viral loads, labelled as underimmunosuppressed, experienced rejection, while none of the overimmunosuppressed patients did. Conversely, the only patient with cytomegalovirus infection was the most overimmunosuppressed patient (TTV load of 10.79 log10 copies/mL). These findings suggest that the combined measurement of dd-cfDNA and TTV viral load could non-invasively identify which patients with molecular damage were underimmunosuppressed and at risk of rejection or overimmunosuppressed and at risk of graft infection. However, our study is underpowered to confirm this hypothesis, so we suggest that new studies including more patients using this dual monitoring should be carried out.

Since the viral load of TTV is a measure of the state of immunosuppression, it is of utmost interest to know what the relationship is between that and the immunosuppressive drugs used in solid organ transplantation. The results of previous studies have provided partially contradictory results. In relation to calcineurin inhibitors (CNIs), some studies detected that patients with higher levels presented a higher viral load [23,24]. However, this finding was not confirmed in other studies [25–32]. In our population of renal transplant recipients, we previously demonstrated the absence of a relationship between TTV viral load and trough levels of tacrolimus, cumulative exposure measured by the mean value of trough levels, the concentration/dose ratio (C/D) of tacrolimus, and two exposure variability markers: the coefficient of variability and time in the therapeutic range [15]. We also did not observe that TTV viral load was related to trough levels of mycophenolic acid or its area under the curve [15]. Rather than being related to levels maintained over time, the viral load seems to be related to changes in immunosuppressants. On the one hand, Regele et al. observed that the reduction in the dose and levels of tacrolimus was associated with a decrease in TTV viral load two months after the dose change, although the increase in dose and levels was not significantly associated with an increase in viral load [33]. On the other hand, Benning et al. and Regele et al. have reported that TTV viral load decreases after the withdrawal of mycophenolic acid [34,35]. It is also not well-known if the increased immunosuppression associated with the treatment of acute rejection modifies the TTV viral load. Reineke et al. have reported that treatment with high-dose corticosteroid pulse therapy as anti-rejection therapy significantly increased the TTV viral load from before the biopsy (median 4.07 log10 copies/mL, IQR 3.22–5.01 log10 copies/mL) to days 30 (median 4.88 log10 copies/mL, IQR 4.06–6.13 log10 copies/mL, $p < 0.005$) and 90 post-treatment (median 5.26 log10 copies/mL, IQR 4.28–7.57 log10 copies/mL, $p < 0.001$) in 31 patients [36]. Our results reflect the evolution of patients treated for antibody-mediated rejection for the first time. The difference in TTV viral load was +6.58 log10 copies/mL in treated patients compared to untreated patients. Although the number of patients was low, our study suggests that treatment with plasmapheresis and IVIg increases the TTV viral load more intensely than treatment with high-dose corticosteroids. In fact, all patients treated for AbMR became overimmunosuppressed and, therefore, at a high risk of infection. This finding should be confirmed in further studies.

In the field of immunosuppressive therapy, the choice of induction therapy has been shown to have a significant impact on the outcome of a kidney transplant. Induction therapy with thymoglobulin has been shown to reduce the risk of acute rejection and increase the risk of developing opportunistic infections, while Basiliximab reduces the occurrence of rejection in the first year [37,38]. In this regard, it is essential to understand how induction therapy influences the TTV viral load and whether it alters the relationship between viral load and both rejection and the risk of infections of significant concern. Various studies have linked receiving induction therapy, or specifically thymoglobulin, with a higher TTV viral load in the first months after solid organ transplantation [15,25,27,32,39–42]. The impairment of T-cell-mediated immunity caused by induction therapy, especially thymoglobulin, appears to favour TTV replication; however, due to the low number of cases, in our study we only found a non-significant trend toward higher viral loads in patients who had received induction. Nevertheless, it was observed that the TTV load and its growth from months one to three were higher in patients who suffered from opportunistic infections beyond the third month and in those who had received therapy for AbMR, respectively, regardless of the use of induction.

Although we did not find a significant relationship between a high TTV load in the first month and the risk of infection, our results showed that the TTV load in the third month was associated with the development of infection. This finding has previously been reported by most, but not all, studies conducted in kidney transplant recipients [15,39–41,43–47]. A meta-analysis including seven studies analysing the performance of the TTV load for infection discrimination in kidney transplant recipients reported that the pooled area under the receiver operating characteristics curve was 0.68, with the TTV load being linearly associated with infection [8]. The Vienna group reported that the TTV load was already lower 1–3 months (27–77 days) before the development of infection [43,44]. In contrast, the absence of a relationship between the TTV load at month one and the development of infections in our study could be due not only to the low number of patients included but also to the low incidence of infectious events between the first and third months.

The present study demonstrated the usefulness of measuring the TTV load to estimate the immunosuppressive status, even in a specific high-risk group of patients with high molecular injury and a high AbMR rate. The study also showed that 'TTV load-defined' overimmunosuppressed kidney transplant recipients had both very high infection and opportunistic infection rates. Consequently, we support the utilisation of the cut-off values proposed by the Vienna group to monitor the immunosuppressive status of kidney transplant recipients at risk, a practice that should be implemented from the first month up to the 12th month of the post-transplantation period [6]. Interestingly, the Lyon group has reported different TTV load thresholds (3.75–5.1 log10 copies/mL) in kidney transplant recipients beyond the first year after transplantation, which were associated with a reduced complication risk. In this study, a TTV load above the upper cut-off was the sole variable independently related (HR 9.41, 95%CI 2.52–35.20) to the risk of infection or cancer as an overimmunosuppression biomarker [48]. We can argue about the usefulness of knowing the net state of immunosuppression in a kidney transplant recipient who has been treated for a previous rejection episode. It is evident that the patient is likely to become overimmunosuppressed following rejection therapy, or alternatively, the rejection-related underimmunosuppressive status is reversed. However, the identification of the overimmunosuppressive status through measuring the TTV load in high-risk patients would facilitate the design of surveillance strategies to detect infection earlier or modify prophylactic therapy. For instance, this could involve prolonging cytomegalovirus prophylaxis beyond the third month only in these patients. These suggestions require confirmation through specifically designed studies.

The limitations of the present study are evident. The sample size is small, the follow-up period is short, and the study is single-centre, which limits the generalisability of the results without larger multicentre prospective studies. However, the study is significant because, for the first time, it performs a joint prospective analysis of two relevant biomarkers that provide complementary information for the follow-up of solid organ transplants.

In conclusion, we have conducted a pioneering study in which we have utilised a dual monitoring approach in kidney transplant recipients, employing biomarkers that offer complementary information. This approach has the potential to enhance post-transplant monitoring. Our methodology involved the use of donor-derived cell-free DNA to identify recipients with greater molecular injury, and TTV load as a metric to assess the overall immunosuppressive status. The results of this study indicated that patients exhibiting molecular damage secondary to rejection tended to be underimmunosuppressed, as indicated by a low TTV load. Following treatment for antibody-mediated rejection, there was a notable increase in TTV load, resulting in a transition from under- to overimmunosuppressed status for all patients. Furthermore, a high TTV load during the third month post-transplant was found to be associated with an elevated risk of opportunistic infections. Of interest, these relationships were independent of exposure to induction therapy. The measurement of TTV load in high-risk patients facilitates the identification of those who are overimmunosuppressed and thus have an increased susceptibility to infection. It is hypothesised that these patients would benefit from the implementation of more rigorous strategies for the early detection of opportunistic infections or alterations in prophylaxis regimens. However, the efficacy of these approaches must be evaluated through the execution of meticulously designed studies.

Author Contributions: Conceptualisation, E.R., J.G.O.-V. and A.B.-H.; methodology, E.R., E.G.-L., J.G.O.-V. and A.B.-H.; software, E.R. and J.G.O.-V.; validation, E.P., C.G.-M., C.L.d.M., A.G.-S. and J.C.R.; formal analysis, E.R. and J.G.O.-V.; investigation, E.R., E.G.-L., J.G.O.-V., A.B.-H. and M.V.F.; resources, E.R., J.G.O.-V. and A.B.-H.; data curation, E.R., E.G.-L., J.G.O.-V. and A.B.-H.; writing—original draft preparation, E.R.; writing—review and editing, E.R., E.G.-L., J.G.O.-V. and A.B.-H.; funding acquisition, E.R., J.G.O.-V. and A.B.-H. All authors have read and agreed to the published version of the manuscript.

Funding: This research was funded by grants for Fondo de Investigaciones Sanitarias-ISCIII (PI20/01710) and RICORS (ISCIII RD21/0005/0010 and RD24/0004/0019, "Financiado por la Unión Europea —NextGenerationEU", Mecanismo para la Recuperación y la Resiliencia [MRR]).

Institutional Review Board Statement: This study was conducted in accordance with the Declaration of Helsinki and approved by the Regional Ethics Committee of Cantabria (reference number: PI20/01710), approval date 22 December 2020.

Informed Consent Statement: Informed consent was obtained from all subjects involved in this study.

Data Availability Statement: The data presented in this study are available on request from the corresponding author.

Acknowledgments: The authors are indebted to Consuelo Agüeros (Nephrology Research Laboratory, Hospital Marqués de Valdecilla-IDIVAL) for technician support.

Conflicts of Interest: The authors declare no conflicts of interest. The funders had no role in the design of this study; in the collection, analyses, or interpretation of data; in the writing of the manuscript; or in the decision to publish the results.

Abbreviations

The following abbreviations are used in this manuscript:

AbMR	antibody-mediated rejection
CMV	cytomegalovirus
dd-cfDNA	donor-derived circulating free DNA
EBV	Epstein–Barr virus
HBV	Hepatitis B virus
HCV	Hepatitis C virus
HSV	Herpes simplex virus
IQR	interquartile range
MPA	mycophenolic acid
KTx	kidney transplant recipients
TTV-load	Torque Teno virus load
VZV	Varicella zoster virus

References

1. Dugast, E.; Soulillou, J.; Foucher, Y.; Papuchon, E.; Guerif, P.; Paul, C.; Riochet, D.; Chesneau, M.; Cesbron, A.; Renaudin, K.; et al. Failure of Calcineurin Inhibitor (Tacrolimus) Weaning Randomized Trial in Long-Term Stable Kidney Transplant Recipients. *Am. J. Transplant.* **2016**, *16*, 3255–3261. [CrossRef]
2. Briggs, J.D. Causes of death after renal transplantation. *Nephrol. Dial. Transplant.* **2001**, *16*, 1545–1549. [CrossRef] [PubMed]
3. Buell, J.F.; Gross, T.G.; Woodle, E.S. Malignancy after transplantation. *Transplantation* **2005**, *80* (Suppl. S2), S254–S264. [CrossRef] [PubMed]

4. Andrews, L.M.; Li, Y.; De Winter, B.C.M.; Shi, Y.Y.; Baan, C.C.; Van Gelder, T.; Hesselink, D.A. Pharmacokinetic considerations related to therapeutic drug monitoring of tacrolimus in kidney transplant patients. *Expert Opin. Drug. Metab. Toxicol.* **2017**, *13*, 1225–1236. [CrossRef] [PubMed]
5. Garcia-Lopez, A.; Calderon-Zapata, A.; Gomez-Montero, A.; Lozano-Suarez, N.; Giron-Luque, F. The Value of Protocol Biopsy in Kidney Transplantation on Monitoring Transplant Outcomes: A Systematic Review and Meta-Analysis. *Transplant. Proc.* **2024**, *56*, 1231–1240. [CrossRef]
6. Jaksch, P.; Görzer, I.; Puchhammer-Stöckl, E.; Bond, G. Integrated Immunologic Monitoring in Solid Organ Transplantation: The Road Toward Torque Teno Virus-guided Immunosuppression. *Transplantation* **2022**, *106*, 1940–1951.
7. Van Rijn, A.L.; Roos, R.; Dekker, F.W.; Rotmans, J.I.; Feltkamp, M. Torque teno virus load as marker of rejection and infection in solid organ transplantation–A systematic review and meta-analysis. *Rev. Med. Virol.* **2023**, *33*, e2393. [CrossRef]
8. Zeng, J.; Tang, Y.; Lin, T.; Song, T. Torque-teno virus for the prediction of graft rejection and infection disease after kidney transplantation: A systematic review and meta-analysis. *J. Med. Virol.* **2023**, *95*, e28677. [CrossRef]
9. Thongprayoon, C.; Vaitla, P.; Craici, I.M.; Leeaphorn, N.; Hansrivijit, P.; Salim, S.A.; Bathini, T.; Rivera, F.H.C.; Cheungpasitporn, W. The Use of Donor-Derived Cell-Free DNA for Assessment of Allograft Rejection and Injury Status. *J. Clin. Med.* **2020**, *9*, 1480. [CrossRef]
10. Wijtvliet, V.P.; Plaeke, P.; Abrams, S.; Hens, N.; Gielis, E.M.; Hellemans, R.; Massart, A.; Hesselink, D.A.; De Winter, B.Y.; Abramowicz, D.; et al. Donor-derived cell-free DNA as a biomarker for rejection after kidney transplantation: A systematic review and meta-analysis. *Transplant. Int.* **2020**, *33*, 1626–1642. [CrossRef]
11. Xing, Y.; Guo, Q.; Wang, C.; Shi, H.; Zheng, J.; Jia, Y.; Li, C.; Hao, C. Donor-derived cell-free DNA as a diagnostic marker for kidney-allograft rejection: A systematic review and meta-analysis. *Biomol. Biomed.* **2024**, *24*, 731. [CrossRef]
12. González-López, E.; Ocejo-Vinyals, J.G.; Renuncio-García, M.; Roa-Bautista, A.; Arribas, D.S.S.; Escagedo, C.; García-Saiz, M.d.M.; Valero, R.; García-Berbel, P.; Millán, J.C.R.S.; et al. Donor-derived cell-free DNA at 1 month after kidney transplantation relates to HLA Class II eplet mismatch load. *Biomed* **2023**, *11*, 2741. [CrossRef]
13. Mayer, K.A.; Omic, H.; Weseslindtner, L.; Doberer, K.; Reindl-Schwaighofer, R.; Viard, T.; Tillgren, A.; Haindl, S.; Casas, S.; Eskandary, F.; et al. Levels of donor-derived cell-free DNA and chemokines in BK polyomavirus-associated nephropathy. *Clin. Transplant.* **2022**, *36*, e14785. [CrossRef]
14. Bloom, R.D.; Bromberg, J.S.; Poggio, E.D.; Bunnapradist, S.; Langone, A.J.; Sood, P.; Matas, A.J.; Mehta, S.; Mannon, R.B.; Sharfuddin, A.; et al. Circulating Donor-Derived Cell-Free DNA in Blood for Diagnosing Active Rejection in Kidney Transplant Recipients (DART) Study Investigators. Cell-Free DNA and Active Rejection in Kidney Allografts. *J. Am. Soc. Nephrol.* **2017**, *28*, 2221–2232. [CrossRef] [PubMed]
15. Cañamero, L.; Benito-Hernández, A.; González, E.; Escagedo, C.; Rodríguez-Vidriales, M.; García-Saiz, M.d.M.; Valero, R.; Belmar, L.; de Cos, M.A.; Francia, M.V.; et al. Torque teno virus load predicts opportunistic infections after kidney transplantation but is not associated with maintenance immunosuppression exposure. *Biomedicines* **2023**, *11*, 1410. [CrossRef] [PubMed]
16. Görzer, I.; Haupenthal, F.; Maggi, F.; Gelas, F.; Kulifaj, D.; Brossault, L.; Puchhammer-Stöckl, E.; Bond, G. Validation of plasma Torque Teno viral load applying a CE-certified PCR for risk stratification of rejection and infection post kidney transplantation. *J. Clin. Virol.* **2023**, *158*, 105348. [CrossRef]
17. Schinstock, C.A.; Mannon, R.B.; Budde, K.; Chong, A.S.; Haas, M.; Knechtle, S.; Lefaucheur, C.; Montgomery, R.A.; Nickerson, P.; Tullius, S.G.; et al. Recommended treatment for antibody-mediated rejection after kidney transplantation: The 2019 expert consensus from the transplantion society working group. *Transplantation* **2020**, *104*, 911–922. [CrossRef]
18. Tharmaraj, D.; Mulley, W.R.; Dendle, C. Current and emerging tools for simultaneous assessment of infection and rejection risk in transplantation. *Front. Immunol.* **2024**, *15*, 1490472. [CrossRef]
19. Kim, H.D.; Bae, H.; Kang, H.; Lee, H.; Eum, S.H.; Yang, C.W.; Choi, Y.J.; Chung, B.H.; Oh, E.-J. Donor-derived cell-free DNA predicted allograft rejection and severe microvascular inflammation in kidney transplant recipients. *Front. Immunol.* **2024**, *15*, 1433918. [CrossRef]
20. Akifova, A.; Budde, K.; Amann, K.; Buettner-Herold, M.; Choi, M.; Oellerich, M.; Beck, J.; Bornemann-Kolatzki, K.; Schütz, E.; Bachmann, F.; et al. Donor-derived cell-free DNA monitoring for early diagnosis of antibody-mediated rejection after kidney transplantation: A randomized trial. *Nephrol. Dial. Transplant.* **2025**, *in press*. [CrossRef]
21. Mayer, K.A.; Schrezenmeier, E.; Diebold, M.; Halloran, P.F.; Schatzl, M.; Schranz, S.; Haindl, S.; Kasbohm, S.; Kainz, A.; Eskandary, F.; et al. A randomized phase 2 trial of felzartamab in antibody-mediated rejection. *N. Eng. J. Med.* **2024**, *391*, 122–132. [CrossRef]
22. Wen, J.; Sun, R.; Yang, H.; Ran, Q.; Hou, Y. Detection of BK polyomavirus-associated nephropathy using plasma graft-derived cell-free DNA: Development of a novel algorithm from programmed monitoring. *Front. Immunol.* **2022**, *13*, 1006970. [CrossRef] [PubMed]

23. Jaksch, P.; Kundi, M.; Görzer, I.; Muraközy, G.; Lambers, C.; Benazzo, A.; Hoetzenecker, K.; Klepetko, W.; Puchhammer-Stöckl, E. Torque teno virus as a novel biomarker targeting the efficacy of immunosuppression after lung transplantation. *J. Infect. Dis.* **2018**, *218*, 1922–1928. [CrossRef] [PubMed]
24. Görzer, I.; Haloschan, M.; Jaksch, P.; Klepetko, W.; Puchhammer-Stöckl, E. Plasma DNA levels of Torque teno virus and immunosuppression after lung transplantation. *J. Heart Lung Transplant.* **2014**, *33*, 320–323. [CrossRef]
25. Görzer, I.; Jaksch, P.; Kundi, M.; Seitz, T.; Klepetko, W.; Puchhammer-Stöckl, E. Pre-transplant plasma Torque Teno virus load and increase dynamics after lung transplantation. *PLoS ONE* **2015**, *10*, e0122975. [CrossRef] [PubMed]
26. Focosi, D.; Macera, L.; Pistello, M.; Maggi, F. Torque Teno virus viremia correlates with intensity of maintenance immunosuppression in adult orthotopic liver transplant. *J. Infect. Dis.* **2014**, *210*, 667–668. [CrossRef]
27. Schiemann, M.; Puchhammer-Stöckl, E.; Eskandary, F.; Kohlbeck, P.; Rasoul-Rockenschaub, S.; Heilos, A.; Kozakowski, N.; Görzer, I.; Kikić, Ž.; Herkner, H.; et al. Torque Teno Virus Load-Inverse Association with Antibody-Mediated Rejection After Kidney Transplantation. *Transplantation* **2017**, *101*, 360–367. [CrossRef]
28. Frye, B.C.; Bierbaum, S.; Falcone, V.; Köhler, T.C.; Gasplmayr, M.; Hettich, I.; Dürk, T.; Idzko, M.; Zissel, G.; Hengel, H.; et al. Kinetics of Torque Teno Virus-DNA Plasma Load Predict Rejection in Lung Transplant Recipients. *Transplantation* **2019**, *103*, 815–822. [CrossRef]
29. Solis, M.; Velay, A.; Gantner, P.; Bausson, J.; Filipputtu, A.; Freitag, R.; Moulin, B.; Caillard, S.; Fafi-Kremer, S. Torqueteno-virus viremia for early prediction of graft rejection after kidney transplantation. *J. Infect.* **2019**, *79*, 56–60. [CrossRef]
30. Ruiz, P.; Martínez-Picola, M.; Santana, M.; Muñoz, J.; Pérez-Del-Pulgar, S.; Koutsoudakis, G.; Sastre, L.; Colmenero, J.; Crespo, G.; Navasa, M. Torque Teno Virus Is Associated with the State of Immune Suppression Early After Liver Transplantation. *Liver Transpl.* **2019**, *25*, 302–310. [CrossRef]
31. Berg, R.; Clemmensen, T.S.; Petersen, M.S.; Mogensen, L.J.; Christiansen, M.; Rolid, K.; Nytrøen, K.; Møller, B.K.; Gullestad, L.; Eiskjær, H.; et al. Kinetics of Torque Teno virus in heart transplant patients. *Human Immunol.* **2023**, *84*, 110720. [CrossRef] [PubMed]
32. Reineke, M.; Speer, C.; Bundschuh, C.; Klein, J.A.F.; Loi, L.; Sommerer, C.; Zeier, M.; Schnitzler, P.; Morath, C.; Benning, L. Impact of induction agents and maintenance immunosuppression on Torque Teno virus loads and year-one complications after kidney transplantation. *Front. Immunol.* **2024**, *13*, 1492611. [CrossRef]
33. Regele, F.; Haupenthal, F.; Doberer, K.; Görzer, I.; Kapps, S.; Strassl, R.; Bond, G. The kinetics of Torque Teno virus plasma load following calcineurin inhibitor dose change in kidney transplant recipients. *J. Med. Virol.* **2024**, *96*, e29554. [CrossRef] [PubMed]
34. Benning, L.; Morath, C.; Kühn, T.; Bartenschlager, M.; Kim, H.; Beimler, J.; Buylaert, M.; Nusshag, C.; Kälble, F.; Reineke, M.; et al. Humoral response to SARS-CoV-2 mRNA vaccination in previous non-responder kidney transplant recipients after short-term withdrawal of mycophenolic acid. *Front. Med.* **2022**, *9*, 958293. [CrossRef]
35. Regele, F.; Heinzel, A.; Hu, K.; Raab, L.; Eskandary, F.; Faé, I.; Zelzer, S.; Böhmig, G.A.; Bond, G.; Fischer, G.; et al. Stopping of Mycophenolic Acid in Kidney Transplant Recipients for 2 Weeks Peri-Vaccination Does Not Increase Response to SARS-CoV-2 Vaccination-A Non-randomized, Controlled Pilot Study. *Front. Med.* **2022**, *9*, 914424. [CrossRef]
36. Reineke, M.; Morath, C.; Speer, C.; Rudek, M.; Bundschuh, C.; Klein, J.A.; Mahler, C.F.; Kälble, F.; Nusshag, C.; Beimler, J.; et al. Dynamics of torque teno virus load in kidney transplant recipients with indication biopsy and therapeutic modifications of immunosuppression. *Front. Med.* **2024**, *11*, 1337367. [CrossRef]
37. Hill, P.; Cross, N.B.; Barnett, A.N.; Palmer, S.C.; Webster, A.C. Polyclonal and monoclonal antibodies for induction therapy in kidney transplant recipients. *Cochrane Database Syst. Rev.* **2017**, *1*, CD004759. [CrossRef]
38. Webster, A.C.; Ruster, L.P.; McGee, R.G.; Matheson, S.L.; Higgins, G.Y.; Willis, N.S.; Chapman, J.R.; Craig, J.C. Interleukin 2 receptor antagonists for kidney transplant recipients. *Cochrane Database Syst. Rev.* **2010**, *2010*, CD003897. [CrossRef]
39. Fernández-Ruiz, M.; Albert, E.; Giménez, E.; Ruiz-Merlo, T.; Parra, P.; López-Medrano, F.; San Juan, R.; Polanco, N.; Andrés, A.; Navarro, D.; et al. Monitoring of alphatorquevirus DNA levels for the prediction of immunosuppression-related complications after kidney transplantation. *Am. J. Transplant.* **2019**, *19*, 1139–1149. [CrossRef]
40. Maggi, F.; Focosi, D.; Statzu, M.; Bianco, G.; Costa, C.; Macera, L.; Spezia, P.G.; Medici, C.; Albert, E.; Navarro, D.; et al. Early post-transplant torquetenovirus viremia predicts cytomegalovirus reactivations in solid organ transplant recipients. *Sci. Rep.* **2018**, *8*, 15490. [CrossRef]
41. Handala, L.; Descamps, V.; Morel, V.; Castelain, S.; François, C.; Duverlie, G.; Helle, F.; Brochot, E. No correlation between Torque Teno virus viral load and BK virus replication after kidney transplantation. *J. Clin. Virol.* **2019**, *116*, 4–6. [CrossRef] [PubMed]
42. Focosi, D.; Macera, L.; Boggi, U.; Nelli, L.C.; Maggi, F. Short-term kinetics of torque teno virus viraemia after induction immunosuppression confirm T lymphocytes as the main replication-competent cells. *J. Gen. Virol.* **2015**, *96 Pt 1*, 115–117. [CrossRef] [PubMed]
43. Strassl, R.; Schiemann, M.; Doberer, K.; Görzer, I.; Puchhammer-Stöckl, E.; Eskandary, F.; Kikić, Ž.; Gualdoni, G.A.; Vossen, M.G.; Rasoul-Rockenschaub, S.; et al. Quantification of Torque Teno Virus Viremia as a Prospective Biomarker for Infectious Disease in Kidney Allograft Recipients. *J. Infect. Dis.* **2018**, *218*, 1191–1199. [CrossRef]

44. Doberer, K.; Schiemann, M.; Strassl, R.; Haupenthal, F.; Dermuth, F.; Görzer, I.; Eskandary, F.; Reindl-Schwaighofer, R.; Kikić, Ž.; Puchhammer-Stöckl, E.; et al. Torque teno virus for risk stratification of graft rejection and infection in kidney transplant recipients—A prospective observational trial. *Am. J. Transplant.* **2020**, *20*, 2081–2090. [CrossRef]
45. Querido, S.; Martins, C.; Gomes, P.; Pessanha, M.A.; Arroz, M.J.; Adragão, T.; Casqueiro, A.; Oliveira, R.; Costa, I.; Azinheira, J.; et al. Kinetics of torque Teno virus viral load is associated with infection and de novo donor specific antibodies in the first year after kidney transplantation: A prospective cohort study. *Viruses* **2023**, *15*, 1464. [CrossRef]
46. Mafi, S.; Essig, M.; Rerolle, J.-P.; Lagathu, G.; Crochette, R.; Brodard, V.; Schvartz, B.; Gouarin, S.; Bouvier, N.; Engelmann, I.; et al. Torque teno virus viremia and QuantiFERON®-CMV assay in prediction of cytomegalovirus reactivation in R+ kidney transplant recipients. *Front. Med.* **2023**, *10*, 1180769. [CrossRef]
47. van Rijn, A.L.; Wunderink, H.F.; Sidorov, I.A.; de Brouwer, C.S.; Kroes, A.C.; Putter, H.; de Vries, A.P.; Rotmans, J.I.; Feltkamp, M.C. Torque teno virus loads after kidney transplantation predict allograft rejection but not viral infection. *J. Clin. Virol.* **2021**, *140*, 104871. [CrossRef]
48. Chauvelot, L.; Barba, T.; Saison, C.; Siska, E.; Kulifaj, D.; Bakker, S.J.L.; Koenig, A.; Rabeyrin, M.; Buron, F.; Picard, C.; et al. Longitudinal monitoring of Torque Teno virus DNAemia in kidney transplant recipients correlates with long-term complications of inadequate immunosuppression. *J. Med. Virol.* **2024**, *96*, e29806. [CrossRef]

Journal of
Clinical Medicine

MDPI

Article

Clinical Factors Influencing Tacrolimus Metabolism and Blood Level Early After Kidney Transplantation—A Comparison of Three Different Tacrolimus Formulations

Aureliusz Kolonko * and Andrzej Więcek

Department of Nephrology, Transplantation and Internal Medicine, Medical University of Silesia, 40-027 Katowice, Poland; awiecek@sum.edu.pl
* Correspondence: uryniusz@wp.pl

Abstract: Background: Optimal tacrolimus dosing in the early post-transplant period is still challenging. We prospectively studied the possible associations between selected parameters of recipient body composition, markers of intestinal permeability and tacrolimus dosing and blood level in kidney transplant recipients (KTRs) treated with three different tacrolimus formulations. **Methods:** When discharged from hospital immediately after kidney transplantation, markers of intestinal permeability, body composition parameters and tacrolimus blood level were assessed in 165 KTRs treated with Prograf, Advagraf or Envarsus. **Results:** In the stepwise multivariate analysis performed in patients treated with Prograf, only age independently influenced the tacrolimus exposure expressed as area under the curve (AUC). In patients treated with Advagraf, eGFR ($r_{partial} = 0.291$; $p < 0.05$), antithymocyte globulin (vs. basiliximab) induction ($r_{partial} = 0.445$; $p < 0.001$), lipopolysaccharide (LPS) level ($r_{partial} = 0.393$; $p < 0.01$) and drug dose ($r_{partial} = 0.433$; $p < 0.01$) were independently associated with tacrolimus AUC. In patients treated with Envarsus, only age ($r_{partial} = -0.365$; $p < 0.05$) and fatty-acid-binding protein (FABP-2) level ($r_{partial} = -0.364$; $p < 0.05$) were independently associated with the tacrolimus AUC. **Conclusions:** We confirmed the significant association between markers of intestinal permeability and tacrolimus exposure in KTRs who underwent early post-transplant conversion from Prograf to Advagraf or Envarsus. This may suggest that the planned tacrolimus conversion from the twice-daily to the once-daily formulation should be performed later (at least 3 months after transplantation) to avoid unnecessary tacrolimus blood level instability.

Keywords: body composition; early conversion; intestinal permeability; tacrolimus formulation

1. Introduction

Today, in a majority of kidney transplant recipients (KTRs), the immunosuppressive regimen is based on tacrolimus. As it is characterized by considerable blood level variability and a narrow therapeutic index, its appropriate dosing is still challenging, especially in the early period after transplantation [1,2]. Moreover, during the last few decades, the innovative once-daily tacrolimus formulations characterized by different mechanisms of drug extended release were successfully introduced. Importantly, these novel tacrolimus formulations present different pharmacokinetics, which makes the precise dosing even more difficult [2–4].

Until now, several clinical factors had been identified as modifying the tacrolimus blood level shortly after transplantation, including recipient age, body mass index (BMI), CYP3A4 polymorphism [5,6], the presence of anti-HCV antibodies [6], hematocrit [7] and comedication [8]. Additionally, the potential relationship between several parameters of body composition and tacrolimus pharmacokinetics was previously investigated [9,10]. In our recent analysis, the pre-transplant lean body mass index (LBMI) assessed by bioimpedance was shown to be a potentially useful tool for the optimization of initial tacrolimus dosing [11].

Finally, it is worth noting that diverse twice-daily and once-daily tacrolimus formulations ex definitione differ substantially in regard to the intestinal absorption site and efficacy [12]. Various disturbances of gastrointestinal tract function, frequently observed during the early post-operative days, significantly modify the intestinal permeability and tacrolimus bioavailability [13]. On the other hand, those disturbances may be further augmented by the immunosuppressive drugs [14]. Furthermore, during the last decade, it was shown that gut microbiota structure could be altered after kidney transplantation and linked to some post-transplant complications, like diarrhea or acute rejection [15]. Importantly, some microbiota species were associated with tacrolimus dosing and exposure in the first post-transplant month [16]. To date, several biomarkers were proposed to assess the intestinal permeability and gut barrier injury, including fatty-acid-binding protein 2 (FABP-2), lipopolysaccharide (LPS), LPS-binding protein (LBP) and zonulin [17–20], although their usefulness is still uncertain. However, both FABP-2 and LPS levels seemed to be reliable measures of intestinal permeability in the KTRs cohort [21].

Based on all the abovementioned evidence, we prospectively investigated the potential associations between recipient body composition parameters, intestinal permeability markers and early post-transplant tacrolimus dosing and exposure in patients treated with three different tacrolimus formulations.

2. Materials and Methods

2.1. Study Group

The analyzed cohort included 165 unselected patients, who were prospectively recruited and studied at the time of cadaveric kidney transplantation in our center. During the first post-transplant hospital stay, patients were divided into three study groups: group 1 (discharged on Prograf®, Astellas Pharma Inc., Chuo City, Japan, n = 56), group 2 (converted to and discharged on Advagraf®, Astellas, n = 59) and group 3 (converted to and discharged on Envarsus®, Chiesi, Parma, Italy, n = 50). In each patient, the tacrolimus exposure was assessed at hospital discharge, using blood trough and 3h post-dose levels, the calculated area under the curve (AUC) and the tacrolimus concentration-to-dose (CD) ratio. On the same day, bioimpedance analysis of body composition was performed. Blood samples were also collected to determine markers of intestinal permeability.

The study was conducted in concordance with the protocol of Helsinki. The Institutional Review Board accepted the study protocol (No KNW/0022/KB1/122/19, BNW/NWN/0052/KB/27/24, accept date: 12 November 2019), and all participants gave written informed consent.

2.2. Immunosuppression Protocol

Before transplantation, all patients received a triple immunosuppressive regimen, which consisted of twice-daily tacrolimus (Prograf), mycophenolate mofetil and steroids. Induction therapy was also prescribed in all subjects, using basiliximab (Simulect®, Novartis, Nurnberg, Germany, n = 105) or antithymocyte globulin (Thymoglobulin®, Genzyme Europe, Naarden, Holland, n = 61). After the second tacrolimus through level measurement, at a median of 8 (7–9) days post-transplant, patients from study groups 2 and 3 were converted in a randomized manner to Advagraf (with the conversion rate 1:1) or Envarsus (with the conversion rate 1:0.7), respectively, whereas patients in group 1 remained on Prograf therapy.

2.3. Bioimpedance Analysis

Body composition analysis was performed on the day of discharge from the hospital using a BIA device (InBody 770, InBody Japan Inc., Tokyo, Japan) with a multifrequency analyzer (1, 5, 50, 500 and 1000 kHz), according to the manufacturer's instructions. Intracellular water (ICW), extracellular water (ECW), total body water (TBW), ECW/TBW ratio, phase angle, visceral fat area (VFA, expressed in cm^2), lean body mass (LBM) and lean body mass index (LBMI, expressed in kg/m^2) were calculated.

2.4. Laboratory Parameters

Plasma levels of IL-6 and bacterial lipopolysaccharides (Uscn Life Sciences Inc., Wuhan, China) were assessed by ELISA, with the intra-assay and inter-assay coefficients of variability <7.2 and <7.8%, and <10 and <12%, respectively. Plasma FABP-2 (R&D systems Inc., Minneapolis, MN, USA) and LBP levels (CloudClone Corp, Katy, TX, USA) were measured by an ELISA kit with the intra-assay and inter-assay coefficients of variability <4.1 and 11.1%, and <10 and <12%, respectively.

2.5. Statistical Analysis

Statistical analyses were performed using Statistica 13.3 PL for Windows (Tibco Inc., Palo Alto, CA, USA) and MedCalc v20.014 (MedCalc Software, Mariakerke, Belgium). Values are presented as means with a 95% confidence interval, medians with interquartile ranges or frequencies. The main study comparison was performed between 3 groups of patients based on different tacrolimus formulations, using the ANOVA (for quantitative variables) or the $\chi 2$ test (for qualitative variables). Variables with a non-normal distribution were compared using the Kruskal–Wallis test. For further between-group comparisons, the Mann–Whitney U-test was used. Calculation of correlations was performed using the Spearman coefficient. Finally, the stepwise multiple regression analyses were performed separately for all three tacrolimus formulations (Prograf, Advagraf and Envarsus) with the tacrolimus AUC at hospital discharge as a dependent variable. The potential independent variables for each multivariate analysis were selected based on the results of univariate analyses. For all analyses, a p value below 0.05 was considered statistically significant.

3. Results

3.1. Study Group Characteristics

The study cohort consisted of 165 kidney transplant recipients, divided into three groups, based on the different tacrolimus formulations (Prograf, Advagraf or Envarsus). The clinical characteristics of study groups are presented in Table 1. There were no significant differences in basic demographic and clinical parameters, including pre-transplant residual diuresis and dialysis vintage. Patients from the Prograf group had a significantly lower BMI and more often received antithymocyte globulin vs. basiliximab induction in comparison with the Advagraf or Envarsus groups. The primary kidney disease diagnosis did not differ between groups ($p = 0.54$). The length of hospital stay [14 (13–18 days)] was also comparable between groups ($p = 0.23$). There were no significant differences in systolic and diastolic blood pressure values and serum creatinine concentration between study groups on the day of the discharge from the hospital.

Table 1. Clinical characteristics of kidney transplant recipients treated with different tacrolimus formulations.

	Prograf N = 56	Advagraf N = 59	Envarsus N = 50	p
		Recipient		
Age [years]	50 (47–53)	50 (47–54)	49 (46–52)	0.88
Sex (M/F)	35/21	35/24	29/21	0.89
BMI * [kg/m^2]	24.2 (21.9–26.6)	25.2 (23.0–29.6)	25.9 (23.3–29.0)	<0.05
Dialysis vintage * [months]	34 (21–55)	33 (21–45)	31 (22–45)	0.71
Residual diuresis * [mL]	300 (25–1000)	500 (100–1500)	500 (100–1200)	0.85
		Transplant procedure		
Donor age * [years]	46.5 (36.5–57.0)	50.0 (39.0–59.0)	50.0 (37.0–57.0)	0.39
Retransplant [%]	19.6	13.6	6.0	0.12
Induction therapy [%]: IL-2 RB ATG	 48.2 51.8	 72.9 27.1	 66.0 34.0	<0.05
CIT [h]	18 (16–19)	17 (15–19)	19 (17–21)	0.22
DGF [%]	16.1	23.7	20.0	0.59
Length of hospital stay [days]	13 (12–15)	14 (13–21) #	15 (13–19) ##	<0.05
		Tacrolimus dosing and exposure		
Tacrolimus daily dose * [mg]	8 (5–10) ^^^	7 (5–11) ^^^	5 (3–7)	<0.001
Tacrolimus dose/kg * [mg/kg]	0.11 (0.08–0.15) ^^^	0.10 (0.07–0.16) ^^^	0.07 (0.04–0.11)	<0.01
Tacrolimus through level * [ng/mL]	9.2 (7.7–11.0)	8.4 (7.2–9.7)	9.3 (7.9–11.6)	0.37
Tacrolimus 3h post-dose level * [ng/mL]	18.2 (16.2–20.3) ^^	20.0 (16.5–22.5) ^^	14.9 (11.4–19.6)	<0.05
Tacrolimus AUC * [ng.h/mL]	149 (137–168)	156 (133–170)	137 (113–171)	0.20
Tacrolimus C/D ratio *	1.20 (0.84–1.68) ^^^	1.17 (0.77–1.70) ^^^	1.93 (1.29–3.00)	<0.001

Data presented as means with 95% confidence interval; * medians with Q1–Q3 values or frequencies, as appropriate. Statistics: ^^ $p < 0.01$, ^^^ $p < 0.001$ vs. the Envarsus group; # $p < 0.05$, ## $p < 0.01$ vs. the Prograf group. BMI, body mass index; IL-2 RB, interleukin-2 receptor blocker; ATG, antithymocyte globulin; CIT, cold ischemia time; DGF, delayed graft function; AUC, area under the curve; C/D, concentration-to-dose.

3.2. Pre-Transplant Factors and Tacrolimus Exposure at Hospital Discharge

As expected, the tacrolimus dosing was significantly lower and the C/D ratio greater in the Envarsus group as compared to the other study groups (Table 1). Importantly, despite the lower 3h post-dose blood level in this group, the discharge tacrolimus AUC was comparable in all three study groups.

In the whole study cohort, the daily dose of tacrolimus (R = −0.332), dose per kg of body weight (R = −0.392) and AUC (R = −0.262) were significantly associated with recipient age (all $p < 0.001$) (Table 2). When study groups were analyzed separately, recipient age was significantly associated with tacrolimus daily dose in both once-daily formulation groups (Advagraf, R = −0.344; $p < 0.01$; Envarsus, R = −0.599; $p < 0.001$) but not in the Prograf group ($p = 0.26$). Moreover, the universal association of recipient age with tacrolimus dose/kg of body weight seems to be much stronger in the Envarsus group (R = −0.603; $p < 0.001$) than in the two other groups (Prograf, R = −0.297; $p < 0.05$; Advagraf, R = −0.397; $p < 0.01$). On the other hand, the AUC was influenced by recipient age in the Prograf group (R = −0.302; $p < 0.05$) and the Advagraf group (R = −0.269; $p < 0.05$) but not in the Envarsus group (Table 2).

Table 2. The associations between recipient age and tacrolimus dosing as well as AUC according to the different tacrolimus formulations.

	Whole Study Group N = 165	Prograf Group N = 56	Advagraf Group N = 59	Envarsus Group N = 50
Tc daily dose [mg]	R = −0.332; $p < 0.001$	NS	R = −0.344; $p < 0.01$	R = −0.599; $p < 0.001$
Tc dose per body kg [mg/kg]	R = −0.392; $p < 0.001$	R = −0.297; $p < 0.01$	R = −0.397; $p < 0.01$	R = −0.603; $p < 0.001$
AUC [ng.h/mL]	R = −0.262; $p < 0.001$	R = −0.302; $p < 0.05$	R = −0.269; $p < 0.05$	NS

Correlations calculated according to Spearman. Tc, tacrolimus; AUC, area under the curve; NS, not significant.

It is of interest that while the amount of pre-transplant residual diuresis or cold ischemia time did not affect the tacrolimus exposure, the time of pre-transplant dialysis therapy was negatively correlated with tacrolimus 3h post-dose level (R = −0.406; $p < 0.01$) and AUC (R = −0.316; $p < 0.05$), but only in the Envarsus group. Similarly, both tacrolimus daily and per-kg dosing (R = −0.460 and R = −0.483, retrospectively; both $p < 0.001$) as well as C/D ratio (R = −0.327; $p < 0.05$) in the latter group were negatively influenced by donor age.

3.3. The Body Composition Parameters and Tacrolimus Dosing and Exposure

No significant differences were found between the study groups in terms of body composition parameters (Table 3).

Table 3. Results of bioimpedance body composition analysis and markers of intestinal permeability at hospital discharge.

	Prograf N = 56	Advagraf N = 59	Envarsus N = 50	p
	Body composition parameters			
Body weight [kg]	71.1 (66.3–74.0)	73.9 (69.6–78.2)	73.7 (69.8–77.7)	0.33
Body fat mass [%]	22.9 (20.5–25.2)	25.5 (23.2–27.9)	25.5 (22.7–28.3)	0.63
ICW * [L]	23.7 (19.5–28.1)	24.5 (20.6–28.1)	24.0 (20.4–28.0)	0.81
ECW * [L]	15.5 (12.6–18.0)	16.4 (13.3–18.4)	15.6 (13.4–17.8)	0.68
ECW/TBW	0.385 (0.391–0.400)	0.384 (0.391–0.399)	0.383 (0.390–0.398)	0.80
Phase angle [°]	4.7 (4.5–5.0)	4.6 (4.4–4.8)	4.8 (4.5–5.1)	0.56
VFA [cm^2] *	84.1 (48.5–104.2)	89.0 (61.8–129.7)	98.8 (56.9–125.5)	0.60
LBM [%]	72.4 (70.2–74.6)	70.1 (67.8–72.3)	70.0 (67.4–72.6)	0.24
LBMI [kg/m^2]	18.3 (17.5–19.1)	18.4 (17.8–19.1)	18.5 (17.8–19.2)	0.95
	Markers of intestinal permeability			
FABP-2 [ng/mL] *	1.8 ^^ (1.1–2.5)	1.4 (0.83–1.9)	1.1 (0.6–1.7)	<0.01
LPS [ng/mL] *	27.8 (23.0–33.2)	28.8 (22.5–38.0)	28.8 (22.5–39.0)	0.75
LBP [μg/mL] *	5.8 ^ (4.9–6.6)	5.1 (3.1–6.6)	4.5 (3.8–6.3)	<0.05
IL-6 [pg/mL] *	5.4 (2.9–8.6) #	3.6 (2.1–5.6)	4.1 (2.6–7.3)	0.1

Data presented as means with a 95% confidence interval; * medians with Q1–Q3 values, as appropriate. Statistics: ^ $p < 0.05$, ^^ $p < 0.01$ vs. the Envarsus group; # $p < 0.05$ vs. the Advagraf group. ICW, intracellular water; ECW, extracellular water; TBW, total body water; VFA, visceral fat area; LBM, lean body mass; LBMI, lean body mass index. FABP-2, intestinal fatty acid binding protein; LPS, lipopolysaccharide; LBP, LPS-binding protein; IL-6, interleukin-6.

As shown in Table 4, the amount of both ECW and ICW positively correlated with tacrolimus daily dose and negatively with the C/D ratio only in the Prograf group, while they correlated negatively with dose per kg in the Advagraf group. Similar relationships were observed for the LBMI. Notably, no such associations were noted in the Envarsus group.

Table 4. The correlations between body composition parameters and tacrolimus exposure measures.

	Daily Dose [mg]	Dose per kg [mg/kg]	Trough Level [ng/mL]	3h Post-Dose Level [ng/mL]	AUC [ng.h/mL]	C/D Ratio
ECW/TBW						
Prograf	-	-	-	R = −0.331; $p < 0.02$	R = −0.340; $p < 0.02$	-
Advagraf	-	-	-	-	-	-
Envarsus	-	-	-	-	-	-
ECW [L]						
Prograf	R = 0.334; $p < 0.02$	-	-	-	-	R = −0.384; $p < 0.01$
Advagraf	-	R = −0.292; $p < 0.05$	-	-	-	-
Envarsus	-	-	-	-	-	-
ICW [L]						
Prograf	R = 0.357; $p < 0.01$	-	-	-	-	R = −0.380; $p < 0.01$
Advagraf	-	R = −0.287; $p < 0.05$	-	-	-	-
Envarsus	-	-	-	-	-	-
LBM [%]						
Prograf	R = 0.267; $p < 0.05$	R = 0.275; $p < 0.05$	-	-	-	R = −0.307; $p < 0.05$
Advagraf	-	R = 0.351; $p < 0.01$	-	-	-	-
Envarsus	-	R = 0.333; $p < 0.02$	-	-	-	-
Phase angle [°]						
Prograf	-	-	-	R = 0.280; $p < 0.05$	R = 0.235; $p = 0.08$	-
Advagraf	-	-	-	-	-	-
Envarsus	R = 0.28; $p < 0.05$	-	-	-	-	-
LBMI [kg/m2]						
Prograf	R = 0.371; $p < 0.01$	-	-	-	-	R = −0.446; $p < 0.001$
Advagraf	-	R = −0.314; $p < 0.02$	-	-	-	-
Envarsus	-	-	-	-	-	-
VFA [cm2]						
Prograf	-	R = −0.347; $p < 0.01$	-	-	-	-
Advagraf	-	R = −0.504; $p < 0.001$	-	-	-	-
Envarsus	R = −0.293; $p < 0.05$	R = −0.453; $p < 0.001$	-	-	-	-

Correlation coefficients calculated according to Spearman. ECW, extracellular water; TBW, total body water; ICW, intracellular water; LBM, lean body mass; LBMI, lean body mass index; VFA, visceral fat area.

In contrast, the percentage of LBM was positively associated with tacrolimus dose per kg in all analyzed groups, while VFA was negatively associated, and these associations were stronger for VFA (Table 4).

Importantly, except the negative influence of the ECW/TBW ratio on the Prograf 3h post-dose level and AUC and the weak positive association of the phase angle on the Prograf 3h post-dose level, any other analyzed body composition parameter did not affect tacrolimus exposure measures (Table 4).

3.4. Markers of Intestinal Permeability and Tacrolimus Exposure

At hospital discharge, median FABP-2 and LBP blood levels were significantly higher in the Prograf group as compared to the Envarsus group (Table 3), whereas median LPS concentrations were comparable in all three study groups.

In the Prograf group, no significant correlation was noted between any analyzed marker of intestinal permeability and neither tacrolimus dosing nor tacrolimus exposure measures. In the Advagraf group, there were weak positive associations between LPS concentration and both tacrolimus 3h level (R = 0.270; $p < 0.05$) and AUC (R = 0.299; $p < 0.05$). In contrast, in the Envarsus group, FABP-2 concentration was significantly negatively associated with tacrolimus exposure (trough: R = −0.296; $p < 0.05$, 3h: R = −0.394; $p < 0.01$, AUC: R = −0.375; $p < 0.01$). Additionally, LPS concentration was significantly positively associated with tacrolimus AUC (R = 0.319; $p < 0.05$).

3.5. The Results of Multivariate Analyses

In the Prograf group, the stepwise multivariate analysis model including recipient age, ECW/TBW ratio and tacrolimus dose showed that only age independently negatively influenced the tacrolimus AUC ($r_{partial} = -0.333$; $p < 0.05$) (with a coefficient of determination R2 value of 0.11).

In the Advagraf group, the initial model included recipient age, eGFR, LPS level, LBP level, tacrolimus dose and the type of induction therapy. The multivariate analysis revealed that eGFR ($r_{partial} = 0.291$; $p < 0.05$), antithymocyte globulin (vs. basiliximab) induction ($r_{partial} = 0.445$; $p < 0.001$), LPS level ($r_{partial} = 0.393$; $p < 0.01$) and tacrolimus dose ($r_{partial} = 0.433$; $p < 0.01$) were independently positively associated with tacrolimus AUC (R2 = 0.39). Notably, an analogic analysis in the homogenous subgroup of patients treated only with basiliximab induction (N = 40) yielded similar results [eGFR ($r_{partial} = 0.526$; $p < 0.001$), LPS level ($r_{partial} = 0.477$; $p < 0.01$) and tacrolimus dose ($r_{partial} = 0.335$; $p < 0.05$)], with the R2 value of 0.45.

In the Envarsus group, the model included recipient age, BMI, tacrolimus dose and FABP-2 level. The multivariate analysis revealed that only age ($r_{partial} = -0.365$; $p < 0.05$) and FABP-2 level ($r_{partial} = -0.364$; $p < 0.05$) were independently negatively associated with the tacrolimus AUC (R2 = 0.22).

3.6. The Tacrolimus Trough Level Variability After Conversion to Once-Daily Formulation

In both conversion groups (Prograf to Advagraf and Prograf to Envarsus group) the drug conversion was performed at a similar post-transplant time [median 8 (7–9) days vs. 8 (7–10) days, respectively; $p = 0.48$]. Prior to conversion, the tacrolimus trough levels (maintained using Prograf formulation) were comparable in both groups [8.9 (6.8–11.2) vs. 8.2 (6.4–11.4) ng/mL, respectively; $p = 0.64$]. Notably, after the conversion, a significantly higher tacrolimus trough level was noted in the Envarsus group 2 days [median 9.9 (7.7–12.5) vs. 8.6 (6.7–10.2) ng/mL; $p < 0.05$] and 4 days [median 9.8 (8.2–13.5) vs. 8.3 (7.1–9.7) ng/mL; $p < 0.01$] after conversion. The percentage of post-conversion tacrolimus trough levels > 11 ng/mL was significantly greater in the Envarsus group than in the Advagraf group, both at day 2 (34 vs. 17%; $p < 0.05$) and day 4 (43.2 vs. 11.4%; $p = 0.001$) post-conversion. Even at hospital discharge, this difference was of borderline significance [median 9.3 (7.9–11.6) vs. 8.4 (7.2–9.7) ng/mL; $p = 0.063$].

4. Discussion

In the present study, we found substantial differences in clinical factors associated with tacrolimus exposure prior to hospital discharge between the groups of patients treated with three different tacrolimus formulations. The analysis comprises demographic and transplant procedure data as well as various recipient body composition parameters and intestinal permeability marker levels. We found that for the twice-daily tacrolimus formulation (Prograf), only the recipient's age influenced the AUC, whereas in the case of both analyzed once-daily formulations, the AUC was also associated with markers of intestinal permeability.

The rationale for such an investigation comes from different pharmacokinetics of all three analyzed drug formulations. Prograf is absorbed mainly in the upper intestine, whereas the tacrolimus granulate formulation (Advagraf) demonstrates prolonged drug release (90% absorption after 6–12 h) [2]. The third formulation, Envarsus, uses the unique MeltDose technique and is characterized by the progressive drug release in the distal intestine [22]. It increases drug bioavailability and decreases drug costs [23] but could also escalate the potential effect of frequently seen disturbances of the gastrointestinal tract function on tacrolimus blood level, which might lead to its excessive variability while using any of the once-daily formulations [24]. Notably, this makes it difficult to promptly achieve and further maintain the target tacrolimus blood concentration and may require more sequential blood level measurements to accomplish this goal. It would be of special importance during the very first post-transplant weeks, as the antibiotics administration was shown to increase the tacrolimus C/D ratio and tacrolimus trough level variability [25].

Moreover, it should be remembered that the uremic milieu itself augments the intestinal permeability in the experimental models [26]; thus, patients with delayed graft function are more prone to the risk of tacrolimus overexposure.

Concisely, in Advagraf-treated patients, the tacrolimus exposure expressed as AUC in both multivariate models was positively modified by eGFR, LPS level and tacrolimus dose, whereas in KTRs receiving Envarsus, only age and FABP-2 negatively influenced the tacrolimus AUC. Taking into account that the LPS level may reflect not only the loss of intestinal epithelium integrity but also the intensity of post-operative inflammation [27], these results do suggest a closer relationship between the intestinal permeability and tacrolimus exposure in the Envarsus-treated patients. Notably, the greater tacrolimus AUC prior to hospital discharge in the patients using antithymocyte globulin versus basiliximab induction probably results from the recent cessation of routine fluconazole prophylaxis in the ATG-treated group.

In our present study, we noticed significant differences in tacrolimus blood levels during the first week post-conversion from twice-daily to once-daily formulation, with inappropriately higher blood levels in the Envarsus group as compared with the Advagraf group, leading to the prolonged time to the target tacrolimus post-conversion level achievement in the former group. This may be a consequence of greater dependence of tacrolimus levels upon the gastrointestinal tract wall injury in Envarsus-treated subjects and may lead to the further exaggeration of bowel disturbances, as the preferential absorption sites were experimentally shown in the proximal and distal tract for Advagraf and Envarsus, respectively [28]. This may also suggest performing early Prograf-to-Envarsus conversion using a lower conversion rate than the one established in the stable patients [29]. However, taking into account that such an early conversion during the first post-transplant weeks requires an adjustment for the improving kidney graft function, fluctuating hemoglobin level, comedication and, of course, non-optimal pre-conversion tacrolimus level, it makes this procedure very complicated, and it would be better to plan it for the following months.

It is worth noting that in the present study, we concurrently investigated several body composition parameters as potential factors influencing tacrolimus exposure, but such an association was not confirmed in the multivariate analysis models. Interestingly, the lean body mass index was previously shown to influence the tacrolimus exposure during the first post-transplant days [11]. Such a discrepancy may suggest that within the first few post-transplant weeks, the frequently observed dysfunction of the gastrointestinal tract as well as the intestinal absorption abnormalities gain the predominant impact on the subsequent tacrolimus exposure, which covers the importance of other possibly relevant factors.

The limitations of the current study include the limited number of participants and the lack of CYP3A5 genotyping. We also did not collect the fecal specimens to determine other markers of intestinal permeability or microbiota.

5. Conclusions

In the present study, we confirmed the significant influence of markers of intestinal permeability on the tacrolimus exposure in KTRs who underwent early post-transplant conversion from Prograf to Advagraf or Envarsus. Taking into account that a substantial percentage of KTRs are supposed to have different disturbances of gastrointestinal tract function during the first post-operative weeks, we believe that the planned conversion of tacrolimus from the twice-daily to the once-daily formulation should be performed later, perhaps from the third month of follow-up, to avoid unnecessary overexposure to tacrolimus and instability of tacrolimus blood levels.

Author Contributions: Conceptualization, A.K. and A.W.; methodology, A.K.; formal analysis, A.K.; investigation, A.K.; data curation, A.K.; writing—original draft preparation, A.K.; writing—review and editing, A.W. All authors have read and agreed to the published version of the manuscript.

Funding: This work was supported by a grant from Medical University of Silesia No BNW-1/089/N/3/K.

Institutional Review Board Statement: The study was conducted in concordance with the protocol of Helsinki. The Institutional Review Board accepted the study protocol (No KNW/0022/KB1/122/19, BNW/NWN/0052/KB/27/24, acceptance date: 12 November 2019).

Informed Consent Statement: Informed consent was obtained from all subjects involved in the study.

Data Availability Statement: The raw data supporting the conclusions of this article will be made available by the authors on request.

Conflicts of Interest: The authors declare no conflicts of interest.

References

1. Bentata, Y. Tacrolimus: 20 years of use in adult kidney transplantation. What we should know about its nephrotoxicity. *Artif. Organs* **2020**, *44*, 140–152. [CrossRef] [PubMed]
2. Henkel, L.; Jehn, U.; Tholking, G.; Reuter, S. Tacrolimus—Why pharmacokinetics matter in the clinic. *Front. Transplant.* **2023**, *21*, 1160752. [CrossRef] [PubMed]
3. Caillard, S.; Moulin, B.; Buron, F.; Mariat, C.; Audard, V.; Grimbert, P.; Marquet, P. Advagraf, a once-daily prolonged release tacrolimus formulation, in kidney transplantation: Literature review and guidelines from a panel of experts. *Transplant. Int.* **2016**, *29*, 860–869. [CrossRef]
4. Tan, T.; Bunnapradist, S. Comparing the pharmacokinetics of extended-relase tacrolimus (LCP-TAC) to immediate-release formulations in kidney transplant patients. *Expert. Opin. Drug Metab. Toxicol.* **2021**, *10*, 1175–1186. [CrossRef]
5. Stratta, P.; Quaglia, M.; Cena, T.; Antoniotti, R.; Fenoglio, R.; Menegotto, A.; Ferrante, D.; Genazzani, A.; Terrazzino, S.; Magnani, C. The interactions of age, sex, body mass index, genetics, and steroid weight-based doses on tacrolimus dosing requirement after adult kidney transplantation. *Eur. J. Clin. Pharmacol.* **2012**, *68*, 671–680. [CrossRef]
6. Krzyżowska, K.; Kolonko, A.; Giza, P.; Chudek, J.; Więcek, A. Which kidney transplant recipients can benefit from the initial tacrolimus dose reduction? *BioMed Res. Int.* **2018**, *2018*, 4573452. [CrossRef]
7. Størset, E.; Holford, N.; Midtvedt, K.; Bremer, S.; Bergan, S.; Asberg, A. Importance of hematocrit for a tacrolimus "target concentration strategy". *Eur. J. Clin. Pharmacol.* **2014**, *70*, 65–77. [CrossRef]
8. Vavic, N.; Rancic, N.; Dragojevic-Simic, V.; Draskovic-Pavlovic, B.; Boonjic, D.; Ignjatovic, L.; Mikov, M. The influence of comedication on tacrolimus blood concentration in patients subjected to kidney transplantation: A retrospective study. *Eur. J. Drug Metabol. Pharmacokinet.* **2014**, *39*, 243–253. [CrossRef]
9. Han, S.S.; Kim, D.H.; Lee, S.M.; Han, N.Y.; Oh, J.M.; Ha, J.; Kim, Y.S. Pharmacokinetics of tacrolimus according to body composition in recipients of kidney transplants. *Kidney Res. Clin. Pract.* **2012**, *31*, 157–162. [CrossRef]
10. Francke, M.I.; Visser, W.J.; Severs, D.; de Mik-van Egmond, A.M.E.; Hesselink, D.A.; De Winter, B.C.M. Body composition is associated with tacrolimus pharmacokinetics in kidney transplant recipients. *Eur. J. Clin. Pharmacol.* **2022**, *78*, 1273–1287. [CrossRef]
11. Kolonko, A.; Pokora, P.; Słabiak-Błaż, N.; Czerwieńska, B.; Karkoszka, H.; Kuczera, P.; Piecha, G.; Więcek, A. The relationship between initial tacrolimus metabolism rate and recipients body composition in kidney transplantation. *J. Clin. Med.* **2021**, *10*, 5793. [CrossRef] [PubMed]
12. Piotti, G.; Cremaschi, E.; Maggiore, U. Once-daily prolonged-release tacrolimus formulations for kidney transplantation: What the nephrologist needs to know. *J. Nephrol.* **2017**, *30*, 53–61. [CrossRef] [PubMed]
13. Vanhove, T.; Annaert, P.; Kuypers, D.R.J. Clinical determinants of calcineurin inhibitor disposition: A mechanistic review. *Drug Metab. Rev.* **2016**, *48*, 88–112. [CrossRef]
14. Bulbuloglu, S.; Gunes, H.; Saritas, S. The effect of long-term immunosuppressive therapy on gastrointestinal symptoms after kidney transplantation. *Transplant. Immunol.* **2022**, *70*, 101515. [CrossRef]
15. Lee, J.R.; Muthukumar, T.; Dadhania, D.; Toussaint, N.C.; Ling, L.; Pamer, E.; Suthanthiran, M. Gut microbiota community structure and complications after kidney transplantation: A pilot study. *Transplantation* **2014**, *98*, 697–705.
16. Lee, J.R.; Muthukumar, T.; Dadhania, D.; Taur, Y.; Jenq, R.R.; Toussaint, N.C.; Ling, L.; Pamer, E.; Suthanthiran, M. Gut microbiota and tacrolimus dosing in kidney transplantation. *PLoS ONE* **2015**, *10*, e0122399. [CrossRef]

17. Terpstra, M.L.; Singh, R.; Geerlings, S.E.; Bemelman, F.J. Measurement of the intestinal permeability in chronic kidney disease. *World J. Nephrol.* **2016**, *5*, 378–388. [CrossRef]
18. Funaoka, H.; Kanda, T.; Fujii, H. Intestinal fatty acid-binding protein (I-FABP) as a new biomarker for intestinal disease. *Rinsho Byori* **2010**, *58*, 162–168.
19. Piton, G.; Capellier, G. Biomarkers of gut barrier failure in the ICU. *Curr. Opin. Crit. Care* **2016**, *22*, 152–160. [CrossRef]
20. Seethaler, B.; Basrai, M.; Neyrinck, A.M.; Nazare, J.-A.; Walter, J.; Delzenne, N.M.; Bischoff, S.C. Biomarkers for assessment of intestinal permeability in clinical practice. *Am. J. Physiol. Gastroinvest. Liver Physiol.* **2021**, *321*, G11–G17. [CrossRef]
21. Kolonko, A.; Słabiak-Błaż, N.; Pokora, P.; Piecha, G.; Więcek, A. Intestinal permeability in patients early after kidney transplantation treated with two different formulations of once-daily tacrolimus. *Int. J. Mol. Sci.* **2023**, *24*, 8344. [CrossRef] [PubMed]
22. Sanchez Fructuoso, A.; Ruiz, J.C.; Franco, A.; Diekmann, F.; Redondo, D.; Calvino, J.; Serra, N.; Aladren, M.J.; Cigarran, S.; Manonelles, A.; et al. Effectiveness and safety of the conversion to MeltDose Extended-release tacrolimus from other formulations of tacrolimus in stable kidney transplant patients: A retrospective study. *Clin. Transplant.* **2020**, *34*, e13767. [CrossRef] [PubMed]
23. Glander, P.; Waiser, J.; Kasbohm, S.; Friedersdorff, F.; Peters, R.; Rudolph, B.; Wu, K.; Budde, K.; Liefeldt, L. Bioavailability and costs of once-daily and twice-daily tacrolimus formulations in de novo kidney transplantation. *Clin. Transplant.* **2018**, *32*, e13311. [CrossRef] [PubMed]
24. Coilly, A.; Calmus, Y.; Chermak, F.; Dumotier, J.; Duvoux, C.; Guillaud, O.; Houssel-Debry, P.; Neau-Cransac, M.; Stocco, J. Once-daily prolonged release tacrolimus in liver transplantation: Experts' literature review and recommendations. *Liver Transplant.* **2015**, *21*, 1312–1321. [CrossRef]
25. Zheng, Y.P.; Masand, A.; Wagner, M.; Kapur, S.; Dadhania, D.; Lubetzky, M.; Lee, J.R. Identification of antibiotic administration as a potential novel factor associated with tacrolimus trough variability in kidney transplant recipients: A preliminary study. *Transplant. Direct* **2019**, *5*, e485. [CrossRef]
26. Vaziri, N.D.; Goshtasbi, N.; Yuan, J.; Jellbauer, S.; Moradi, H.; Rafatellu, M.; Kalantar-Zadeh, K. Uremic plasma impairs barrier function and depletes the tight junction protein constituents of intestinal epithelium. *Am. J. Nephrol.* **2012**, *36*, 438–443. [CrossRef]
27. Carron, C.; Pais de Barros, J.-P.; Gaiffe, E.; Deckert, V.; Adda-Rezig, H.; Roubiou, C.; Laheurte, C.; Masson, D.; Simula-Faivre, D.; Louvat, P.; et al. End-stage renal disease-associated gut bacterial translocation: Evolution and impact on chronic inflammation and acute rejection after renal transplantation. *Front. Immunol.* **2019**, *10*, 1630. [CrossRef]
28. Mercuri, A.; Wu, S.; Stranzinger, S.; Mohr, S.; Salar-Behzadi, S.; Bresciani, M.; Frohlich, E. In vitro and in silico characterization of tacrolimus released under biorelevant conditions. *Int. J. Pharm.* **2016**, *515*, 271–280. [CrossRef]
29. Tremblay, S.; Nigro, V.; Weinberg, J.; Woodle, E.S.; Alloway, R.R. A steady-state head-to-head pharmacokinetic comparison of all FK-506 (tacrolimus) formulations (ASTCOFF): An open-label, prospective, randomized, two-arm, three-period crossover study. *Am. J. Transplant.* **2017**, *17*, 432–444. [CrossRef]

Journal of
Clinical Medicine

MDPI

Article

Long-Term Outcomes of Living Kidney Donors Left with Multiple Renal Arteries: A Retrospective Cohort Study from a Single Center

Thomas Kurz, Jacob Schmidt, Isabel Lichy, Irena Goranova, Jonathan Jeutner, Nadine Biernath, Lukas Kurz, Thorsten Schlomm, Robert Peters, Frank Friedersdorff, Henning Plage † and Bernhard Ralla *,†

Charité—Universitätsmedizin Berlin, Corporate Member of Freie Universität Berlin and Humboldt—Universität zu Berlin, Department of Urology, Charitéplatz 1, 10117 Berlin, Germany; thomas.kurz@helios-gesundheit.de (T.K.); till-jacob-valentin.schmidt@charite.de (J.S.); isabel-michaela.lichy@charite.de (I.L.); irena.goranova@charite.de (I.G.); jonathan.jeutner@charite.de (J.J.); nadine.biernath@charite.de (N.B.); lukas.kurz@charite.de (L.K.); thorsten.schlomm@charite.de (T.S.); robert.peters@charite.de (R.P.); frank.friedersdorff@charite.de (F.F.); henning.plage@charite.de (H.P.)

* Correspondence: bernhard.ralla@charite.de

† These authors contributed equally to this work.

Abstract: Background: The presence of multiple renal arteries (MRAs) is a common anatomical variant in living kidney donors. While MRAs are not considered a contraindication to donation, it remains uncertain whether leaving the donor with a kidney containing MRAs affects long-term outcomes. This study aimed to evaluate renal and clinical outcomes in donors based on the vascular anatomy of the remnant kidney. **Methods:** We conducted a retrospective cohort study of living kidney donors who underwent nephrectomy at our institution between 2011 and 2016. Donors were categorized according to the vascular anatomy of the remaining kidney: single renal artery (SRA) vs. multiple renal arteries (MRAs). Data on renal function, hypertension, diabetes mellitus, and cardiovascular events were collected at baseline and follow-up. The primary outcome was long-term renal function, which was measured by the estimated glomerular filtration rate (eGFR). Secondary outcomes included clinical comorbidities and postoperative complications. **Results:** Among 190 donors, 132 had a remaining kidney with a single artery and 58 had MRAs. Over a median follow-up of 89.5 months (SRA) and 74.5 months (MRA), there were no significant differences in eGFR (SRA: 66 mL/min vs. MRA: 65 mL/min, $p = 0.60$), serum creatinine ($p = 0.86$), or the incidence of hypertension (31.8% vs. 34.5%, $p = 0.35$). Rates of diabetes mellitus and cardiovascular events were similarly low and comparable between groups. **Conclusions:** Living kidney donors left with a remnant kidney containing multiple renal arteries have similar long-term renal function and clinical outcomes as those with a single renal artery. These findings support the feasibility of MRA retention in donor selection and contribute to evidence-based surgical planning and donor counseling.

Keywords: living kidney donation; multiple renal arteries; donor nephrectomy; renal function; hypertension; vascular anatomy

1. Introduction

Living kidney donation represents the optimal treatment for many patients with end-stage renal disease, providing superior graft survival, reduced waiting times, and better quality of life compared to deceased donor transplantation [1,2]. As donor eligibility criteria broaden to meet increasing demand, anatomical variations—such as the presence of multiple renal arteries (MRAs)—are being encountered more frequently during routine pre-donation imaging with a reported prevalence of up to 30% [3].

The presence of MRAs has historically raised concerns in both donor nephrectomy and transplantation, which is primarily due to potential technical challenges and postoperative complications [4,5]. In recipients, MRAs may be associated with prolonged operative time, increased ischemia, and a higher risk of vascular or ureteral complications [6]. Kok et al. reported that laparoscopic donor nephrectomies involving MRAs were longer in duration with accessory lower pole arteries contributing to a higher rate of ureteral complications [7]. Mahajan et al. similarly noted extended ischemia and operative times in MRA transplants, although one-year graft and patient survival remained comparable to single-artery transplants [8]. Ghazanfar et al. found a modest increase in acute tubular necrosis and vascular complications in recipients of MRA grafts yet no significant differences in long-term outcomes [9]. Overall, these studies support the clinical safety of MRA grafts, contributing to their broader acceptance in transplantation practice.

As the use of MRA grafts becomes routine, a related but less studied question has emerged: does retaining the kidney with multiple arteries in the donor carry any additional long-term risk? Traditionally, donor nephrectomy is guided by split renal function and surgical accessibility, often leaving the donor with the anatomically more complex kidney when both kidneys have similar function. With increased acceptance of complex anatomy in living donor programs, clarifying this risk is important for informed consent and surgical planning.

Although theoretical mechanisms have proposed that MRAs could contribute to segmental perfusion deficits or altered hemodynamics in the remnant kidney, leading to renovascular hypertension, the clinical relevance of this concern remains debated [10]. Some anatomical and imaging studies suggest that MRAs may be associated with a higher prevalence of hypertension or elevated blood pressure. For example, Glodny et al. reported increased plasma renin activity in individuals with MRAs, which could contribute to the development of hypertension [11]. However, other studies have not demonstrated a consistent association. Earlier investigations by Geyer and Poutasse [12], Bönner et al. [13], and Nomura et al. [14] found no significant difference in MRA frequency between hypertensive and normotensive individuals. More recent data from Gandhi et al., based on a large donor cohort, also showed no increased risk of hypertension or renal complications in normotensive donors with MRAs [15]. Taken together, these findings illustrate the uncertainty surrounding the physiological implications of MRAs and highlight the need for more definitive outcome-based research in living donors.

In this study, we sought to evaluate the long-term renal and clinical outcomes of living kidney donors left with a remnant kidney containing multiple renal arteries. By comparing donors with MRAs in the remaining kidney to those with single renal arteries (SRAs), we aimed to clarify whether remnant vascular anatomy is associated with differences in kidney function, hypertension, or other clinical endpoints during long-term follow-up.

2. Materials and Methods

2.1. Study Design and Population

We performed a retrospective observational cohort study of all living kidney donors who underwent donor nephrectomy at our tertiary academic center between January 2011 and December 2016. Inclusion criteria were as follows: age $\geq$ 18 years at the time of donation, complete documentation of renal vascular anatomy based on preoperative imaging, and availability of follow-up data for renal function and blood pressure. Donors were categorized into two groups based on the vascular anatomy of the remaining kidney: those with a single renal artery (SRA) and those with multiple renal arteries (MRAs).

2.2. Data Collection

Baseline demographic and clinical data were extracted from institutional electronic health records. Renal vascular anatomy was assessed using preoperative contrast-enhanced computed tomography (CT) or magnetic resonance (MR) angiography. Operative and perioperative data were retrieved from surgical reports. The side of donor nephrectomy was determined according to institutional surgical protocol, which prioritizes split renal function. When both kidneys were functionally equivalent, the kidney with a single artery was preferentially selected for removal, and the left kidney was generally favored due to anatomical advantages for transplantation. Postoperative follow-up data were collected from routine outpatient visits, telephone interviews, and general practitioner reports where applicable.

Renal function was assessed using the estimated glomerular filtration rate (eGFR), which was calculated by the CKD–EPI formula. Blood pressure measurements were taken during scheduled follow-ups; hypertension was defined according to the 2018 European Society of Cardiology (ESC) guidelines [16]. Additional comorbidities such as diabetes mellitus, cardiovascular events (myocardial infarction, stroke), and need for renal replacement therapy were recorded. Postoperative complications were classified using the Clavien–Dindo grading system.

2.3. Follow-Up and Outcome Measures

The primary outcome was long-term renal function, which was assessed by the eGFR at last follow-up. Secondary outcomes included incidence of arterial hypertension, new-onset diabetes mellitus, cardiovascular events, and need for dialysis. Clinical follow-up was typically conducted at 3 months, 1 year, and then annually.

2.4. Statistical Analysis

Continuous variables were tested for normality using the Shapiro–Wilk test. Normally distributed variables were compared between groups using the independent-samples *t*-test, whereas non-normally distributed variables were analyzed with the Mann–Whitney U test. Continuous variables are presented as medians with interquartile ranges (IQRs). Categorical variables were analyzed using the chi-square test or Fisher's exact test as appropriate. Multivariable analyses were performed to explore the association of group status (SRA vs. MRA) and other confounding variables (age, BMI, gender, operative time, remnant side, preoperative GFR, follow up, and relevant pre-existing conditions) with continuous outcomes (eGFR at last follow-up) using linear regression and with binary outcomes (presence of hypertension during follow-up) using binary logistic regression. A two-sided p-value < 0.05 was considered statistically significant. To account for multiple comparisons within each outcome table, p-values were adjusted using the Bonferroni correction, and adjusted α-levels were reported accordingly.

Given the smaller size of the MRA group (n = 58) compared to the SRA group (n = 132), a post hoc power analysis was conducted for the two main outcomes: the eGFR at last follow-up and the prevalence of hypertension. The analysis was performed in R using the pwr package. For the eGFR, Cohen's d was calculated, and statistical power and minimal detectable effect size (MDE) were determined. For hypertension, Cohen's h was used to assess power for detecting differences in proportions. Details are provided in Supplementary Table S3.

All statistical analyses were performed using IBM SPSS Statistics for Windows, Version 27.0 (IBM Corp., Armonk, NY, USA) or RStudio 2025.05 (Posit Software, Boston, MA, USA).

3. Results

A total of 190 living kidney donors were included in the study: 132 donors had a remnant kidney with a single renal artery (SRA group), and 58 donors had multiple renal arteries (MRA group). Median follow-up was 89.5 months (IQR 39–124) in the SRA group and 74.5 months (IQR 34–116) in the MRA group.

3.1. Baseline Characteristics

Baseline demographics and preoperative characteristics were comparable between groups, as shown in Table 1. There were no significant differences in age (SRA: 51.0 ± 10.6 years; MRA: 51.8 ± 10.2 years), sex distribution (SRA: 55.3% female; MRA: 48.3% female), or BMI (SRA: 25.3 ± 3.3 kg/m^2; MRA: 25.9 ± 3.4 kg/m^2). Pre-donation kidney function (eGFR) and blood pressure values did not differ significantly.

Table 1. Demographic and patient characteristics.

Characteristics	SRA (n = 132)	MRA (n = 58)	p-Value
Age at transplantation (years)	51.5 (21–58)	52.5 (28–70)	0.75
BMI (kg/m^2)	26.2 (17.6–36.1)	25.1 (17.9–34.5)	0.30
Remnant side			0.34
Left	26 (19.7%)	15 (25.9%)	
Right	106 (80.3%)	43 (74.1%)	
Number of renal arteries in extracted side			0.02
SRA	114 (86.4%)	42 (72.4%)	
MRA	18 (13.6%)	16 (27.6%)	
Left (single/multiple arteries)	91 (85.8%)/15 (14.2%)	28 (66.7%)/14 (33.3%)	
Right (single/multiple arteries)	23 (83.3%)/3 (16.7%)	15 (93.7%/1 (6.3%)	
Operative time (min)	213 (135–333)	224 (120–392)	0.70
Pre-existing medical condition			
Autoimmune disease	6 (4.5%)	3 (5.2%)	0.85 †
Gynecologic disease	14 (10.6%)	4 (6.9%)	0.16 †
Psychiatric disease	5 (3.8%)	3 (5.2%)	0.66 †
Neurologic disease	4 (3.0%)	3 (5.2%)	0.47 †
Orthopedic disease	2 (1.5%)	0	0.35 †
Gastroenterological disease	12 (9.1%)	6 (10.3%)	0.79 †
Dermatologic disease	0	2 (3.4%)	0.03 † (ns)
Struma nodosa	3 (2.3%)	1 (1.7%)	0.81 †
Hypothyroidism	12 (9.1%)	3 (5.2%)	0.36 †
Hyperthyroidism	1 (0.8%)	1 (1.7%)	0.55 †
Hyperlipidemia	12 (9.1%)	9 (15.5%)	0.19 †
Diabetes mellitus	3 (2.3%)	0	0.25 †
Adrenal adenoma	2 (1.5%)	0	0.35 †
Hemostasis disorder	8 (6.1%)	3 (5.2%)	0.81 †
Kidney cysts	9 (6.8%)	5 (8.6%)	0.66 †
Bronchial asthma	5 (3.8%)	2 (3.4%)	0.91 †
COPD	1 (0.8%)	0	0.51 †
Cardiologic disease	8 (6.1%)	1 (1.7%)	0.20 †
Arterial hypertension	27 (20.5%)	13 (22.4%)	0.76 †

Values are shown as median (range) or number (percentage of the group); p-value < 0.05 in t-test, Mann–Whitney U- or Chi-square test.† p-values were adjusted for multiple comparisons using the Bonferroni method (adjusted α = 0.0026). Values that were significant before adjustment but not after correction are indicated with "ns" (not significant).

3.2. Distribution of Arterial Anatomy in Extracted Kidneys

The vascular anatomy of the extracted kidneys was analyzed in relation to nephrectomy side and remnant kidney arterial anatomy. In the SRA group, 91 left kidneys (85.8%)

and 23 right kidneys (88.5%) had a single artery, while 15 left kidneys (14.2%) and 3 right kidneys (11.5%) had multiple arteries. In the MRA group, 28 left kidneys (66.7%) and 15 right kidneys (93.7%) had a single artery, while 14 left kidneys (33.3%) and 1 right kidney (6.3%) had multiple arteries.

A significant difference was observed in left-sided nephrectomies with extracted kidneys showing a higher rate of multiple arteries in the MRA group compared to the SRA group (33.3% vs. 14.2%, $p = 0.02$). No significant difference was found for right-sided nephrectomies (11.5% vs. 6.3%, $p = 0.61$).

3.3. Perioperative Outcomes

Operative parameters including the total operative time, warm ischemia time, and blood loss were similar between the two groups. Intraoperative complications occurred at a low and comparable rate (SRA: 3.1%; MRA: 3.4%; $p = 0.93$). No donor required intraoperative transfusion.

Postoperative complication rates showed some differences: hospital readmissions were more frequent in the MRA group (12.1% vs. 4.5%, $p = 0.07$), and incisional hernias occurred exclusively in MRA donors (3.4% vs. 0%, $p = 0.03$). Postoperative infection was also observed only in MRA donors (5.2%, $p = 0.008$). These infections included two microbiologically confirmed urinary tract infections and one wound infection, which were all occurring in the early postoperative period. No systemic infections or sepsis were recorded. One donor in the MRA group required dialysis during follow-up (Table 2).

Table 2. Perioperative outcome.

Characteristics	SRA (n = 132)	MRA (n = 58)	*p*-Value
Intraoperative complication	4 (3.1%)	2 (3.4%)	0.90
Obstructive vesicoureteral anastomosis	1 (0.8%)	0	
Injury to donor kidney	2 (1.5%)	0	
Splenic lesion	1 (0.8%)	0	
Injury to mesentery of the colon	0	1 (1.7%)	
Conversion due to bleeding	0	1 (1.7%)	
Clavien–Dindo (clinical course)			0.67
II	1 (0.8%)	0	
IIIb	1 (0.8%)	1 (1.7%)	
Hospital readmission	6 (4.5%)	7 (12.1%)	0.06
Reason for readmission			
Hydrocele testis	0	1 (1.7%)	0.13 †
Varicocele testis	0	1 (1.7%)	0.13 †
Incisional hernia	0	2 (3.4%)	0.03 † (ns)
Inguinal hernia	0	1 (1.7%)	0.13 †
Femoral hernia	0	1 (1.7%)	0.13 †
Epididymitis	1 (0.8%)	1 (1.7%)	0.54 †
Acute kidney injury	1 (0.8%)	0	0.51 †
Postoperative hematoma	1 (0.8%)	1 (1.7%)	0.55 †
Acute postoperative bleeding	0	1 (1.7%)	0.13 †
Pancreatitis	1 (0.8%)	0	0.51 †
Chylous ascites	0	1 (1.7%)	0.13 †
Acute hypertensive crisis	0	1 (1.7%)	0.13 †
Paresthesia	1 (0.8%)	0	0.51 †
LUTS	1 (0.8%)	0	0.51 †

Values are shown as median (range) or number (percentage of the group); p-value < 0.05 in Mann–Whitney U-test or Chi-square test.† p-values were adjusted for multiple comparisons using the Bonferroni method (adjusted $\alpha = 0.0036$). Values that were significant before adjustment but not after correction are indicated with "ns" (not significant).

3.4. Postoperative Medical Conditions During Follow-Up

Long-term follow-up revealed no significant differences in the incidence of arterial hypertension (SRA: 31.8%; MRA: 34.5%, $p = 0.35$, Table 3). Cardiovascular and neurological events were rare and did not differ between groups. No donor in either group developed new-onset diabetes mellitus.

Table 3. Postoperative medical condition during follow up.

Characteristics	SRA (n = 132)	MRA (n = 58)	p-Value
Follow up (months)	89.5 (5–158)	74.5 (3–163)	0.96
Infection	0	3 (5.2%)	0.008 † (ns)
Vascular/cardiovascular disease	15 (11.4%)	5 (8.6%)	0.57 †
Malignancy	6 (4.5%)	4 (6.9%)	0.50 †
Neurological/psychiatric disease	10 (7.6%)	3 (5.2%)	0.55 †
Lung disease	3 (2.3%)	1 (1.7%)	0.80 †
Hematological disease/anemia	12 (9.1%)	4 (6.9%)	0.62 †
Incisional hernia or paresthesia/pain	8 (6.1%)	5 (38.5%)	0.52 †
Arterial hypertension (ESC 2018)	42 (31.8%)	20 (34.5%)	0.35
I	30 (23.8%)	19 (33.9%)	
II	5 (4%)	1 (1.8%)	
III	1 (0.8%)	0	
Fatigue symptoms	14 (11.7%)	5 (10%)	0.75 †
Hba1c ≥ 6.5%	18 (13.6%)	3 (5.2%)	0.19 †
Dialysis	0	1 (1.7%)	0.13 †
Albuminuria	32 (24.2%)	13 (22.4%)	0.64 †
Hyperlipidemia	30 (22.7%)	16 (27.6%)	0.47 †

Values are shown as median (range) or number (percentage of the group); p-value < 0.05 in Mann–Whitney U-test or Chi-square test. † p-values were adjusted for multiple comparisons using the Bonferroni method (adjusted $\alpha = 0.0042$). Values that were significant before adjustment but not after correction are indicated with "ns" (not significant).

Mild albuminuria was noted in both groups (SRA: 6.1%; MRA: 6.9%), and one case of macroalbuminuria occurred in the SRA group. There were no differences in rates of hematuria, hyperuricemia, or new malignancy. One donor in the SRA group developed renal stones. Infections requiring hospitalization were significantly more frequent in the MRA group (5.2% vs. 0%, $p = 0.008$), but this finding also did not retain significance after correction (adjusted $\alpha = 0.0042$).

3.5. Renal Function and Comorbidities

Median follow-up was 89.5 months in the SRA group and 74.5 months in the MRA group. The eGFR remained stable and comparable between groups at all time points. At final follow-up, the median eGFR was 66 mL/min (SRA) vs. 65 mL/min (MRA), $p = 0.60$.

Hypertension developed in 31.8% of SRA donors and 34.5% of MRA donors ($p = 0.35$). Kaplan–Meier analysis confirmed no significant difference in time to hypertension diagnosis. Rates of diabetes, albuminuria, and cardiovascular disease were also comparable. One MRA donor required dialysis eight years after donation due to ischemic nephropathy in a polar segment. Infections (UTI or pneumonia) were more frequent in the MRA group (5.2%, $p = 0.008$), but no common etiology was identified. In multivariable analyses, linear regression did not identify a statistically significant association between the presence of MRA, age, BMI, gender, operative time, remnant side, preoperative GFR, follow-up, and relevant pre-existing conditions and the eGFR at last follow-up (Supplementary Table S1). Logistic regression showed no statistically significant association between the mentioned parameters and the presence of hypertension during follow-up (Supplementary Table S2).

3.6. Postoperative Laboratory Parameters at Follow-Up

Laboratory values obtained at the most recent follow-up showed no clinically relevant differences (Table 4). The median serum creatinine was slightly higher in the MRA group (1.08 mg/dL vs. 1.04 mg/dL), while the eGFR values were similar (MRA: 65 mL/min vs. SRA: 66 mL/min, $p = 0.60$). Hemoglobin and hematocrit values were comparable between groups, as were serum albumin and CRP concentrations. The distribution of CKD stages (mostly CKD G2) was not significantly different.

Table 4. Kidney function during follow up.

Characteristics	SRA (n = 132)	MRA (n = 58)	*p*-Value
Follow up (months)	89.5 (5–158)	74.5 (3–163)	0.96
Glomerular filtration rate (GFR) (mL/min)			
Preoperative (DTPA)	119 (85–235)	124.2 (76–237)	0.23
At discharge (eGFR)	57 (38–90)	65 (42–90)	0.98 †
1 month (eGFR)	61 (38–97)	62 (44–90)	0.61 †
6 months (eGFR)	62 (38–92)	58.5 (43–84)	0.07 †
1 year (eGFR)	62.5 (37–124)	59 (45–90)	0.96 †
2 years (eGFR)	66 (39–90)	64 (48–90)	0.59 †
3 years (eGFR)	64 (38–90)	66 (49–90)	0.27 †
4 years (eGFR)	64 (36–90)	63 (42–90)	0.96 †
5 years (eGFR)	66 (39–95)	65 (53–90)	0.36 †
At follow up (eGFR)	66 (38–113)	65 (42–90)	0.55 †
Serum creatinine (mg/dL)			
Preoperative	0.78 (0.49–1.17)	0.77 (0.58–1.37)	0.68 †
At discharge	1.25 (0.64–1.77)	1.16 (0.76–2.01)	0.46 †
At follow up	1.05 (0.66–1.80)	1.03 (0.67–1.67)	0.67 †
CKD at follow up			0.09
I (eGFR 60–89 mL/min)	57 (33.1%)	37 (21.5%)	
II (eGFR 45–59 mL/min)	36 (20.9%)	17 (9.9%)	
III (eGFR 30–44 mL/min)	9 (5.2%)	0	

Values are shown as median (range) or number (percentage of the group); p-value < 0.05 in t-test, Mann–Whitney U- or Chi-square test. † p-values were adjusted for multiple comparisons using the Bonferroni method (adjusted $\alpha = 0.0038$).

3.7. Post-Hoc Power Analysis

For the eGFR at last follow-up, a Cohen's d of −0.098 was observed. The calculated power for this difference was 0.10. For hypertension, a Cohen's h of 0.077 and a calculated power of 0.08 was observed. Based on the current sample sizes, the minimal detectable difference (MDE) for 80% power was 6.4 mL/min/1.73 m^2 for the eGFR and ±20 percentage points for hypertension (Supplementary Tables S3 and S4).

4. Discussion

Our findings confirm that living kidney donors left with a remnant kidney containing MRAs exhibit long-term renal and clinical outcomes comparable to those left with SRAs. Across a median follow-up of over six years, there were no statistically significant differences between groups regarding the eGFR, serum creatinine, incidence of hypertension, or the development of comorbidities.

At final follow-up, the eGFR remained stable and similar in both groups (SRA: 66 mL/min vs. MRA: 65 mL/min, $p = 0.60$), and serum creatinine levels did not differ ($p = 0.86$). Hypertension occurred in 31.8% of SRA and 34.5% of MRA donors ($p = 0.35$) with no significant difference in time to onset in Kaplan–Meier analysis. Similarly, albuminuria rates (SRA: 24.2% vs. MRA: 22.4%) and other metabolic and cardiovascular outcomes were comparable. One MRA donor required dialysis due to localized ischemic nephropathy in a polar segment.

These findings remained robust in multivariate regression analysis adjusting for potential confounding variables, including age, BMI, gender, preoperative GFR, operative time, remnant side, and follow-up duration. MRA status was not significantly associated with either long-term eGFR or the development of hypertension. This supports the notion that vascular anatomy alone does not adversely affect long-term donor outcomes when appropriate donor selection criteria are applied.

Our results align with prior large-scale studies such as Gandhi et al. [15], who examined over 5000 donors and found no association between renal artery anatomy and long-term renal function, hypertension, or cardiovascular events. Similarly, Fehrman-Ekholm et al. [17] and Rizzari et al. [18] reported equivalent donor outcomes in Swedish and North American cohorts, respectively, reinforcing the generalizability of our findings.

Perioperative outcomes were also largely comparable. Although postoperative complications like incisional hernias (3.4%, $p = 0.03$) and infections (5.2%, $p = 0.008$) occurred more frequently in MRA donors, intraoperative complications and overall morbidity were low. These findings are likely multifactorial and not directly attributable to arterial anatomy. Increased vascular complexity may contribute indirectly by prolonging operative time or requiring more extensive dissection. Similar observations were made by Carter et al. [6] and Choi et al. [19], who reported longer warm ischemia times in MRA nephrectomies without associated functional decline.

These observations are consistent with reports by Seet et al. [20], Afshari et al. [21], and Şahin et al. [22], who found that MRAs were associated with increased surgical complexity—such as longer operative or ischemia times—and a slightly higher incidence of early technical complications. However, these did not translate into worse long-term outcomes or increased donor morbidity.

The longstanding concern that MRAs might predispose to segmental hypoperfusion and renovascular hypertension remains largely theoretical. Although systematic perfusion imaging was not performed in our cohort, we found no clinical evidence of functional impairment or elevated risk of hypertension attributable to MRAs. This is consistent with data from Glodny et al. [11], who reported higher plasma renin activity in MRA donors, and Shabalin et al. [23], who found that renovascular hypertension occurred only when one or more arteries were anatomically or functionally compromised. Likewise, large series such as those by Benedetti et al. [24] and Ali-El-Dein et al. [25] found no long-term renal dysfunction in recipients of MRA grafts even when early surgical challenges were encountered.

When stratified by side of nephrectomy, extracted left kidneys showed a significantly higher rate of multiple arteries in the MRA group compared to the SRA group (33.3% vs. 14.2%, $p = 0.02$), whereas no difference was observed in right-sided nephrectomies ($p = 0.61$). This distribution reflects the surgical protocol of selecting the nephrectomy side based primarily on split renal function. When both kidneys are functionally equivalent, the kidney with a single artery is preferentially selected for removal, and the left side is generally favored due to anatomical advantages for transplantation. As a result, donors in the MRA group were more likely to retain kidneys with more complex vascular anatomy without adverse long-term outcomes.

In line with the emerging literature, general anatomical complexity—such as the number or branching pattern of arteries—is not a reliable predictor of long-term function. Specifically, differential renal function and DMSA-based assessments were not associated with the eGFR decline in recent donor cohorts [26]. Instead, studies suggest that remnant cortical volume, as assessed by CT or AI-based tools, may better predict post-donation renal outcomes, especially in older donors [27,28]. Although these methods were not available in our retrospective dataset, they warrant consideration for future prospective studies. Similarly, while early post-donation morphological changes such as compensatory hypertrophy have been described [29], they have not been shown to result in long-term functional decline.

The retrospective design and relatively small sample size, particularly in the MRA group, limit the ability to detect smaller differences or rare events. Importantly, the study was not designed to test equivalence or non-inferiority between groups, and the post hoc power analysis revealed limited statistical power for detecting smaller differences in key outcomes (e.g., 10% for the eGFR and 8% for hypertension). Therefore, while no statistically significant differences were observed, these findings should not be interpreted as evidence of equivalence or comparability between groups. The lack of routine perfusion imaging and reliance on single-center data may also limit generalizability.

Despite these limitations, our findings provide meaningful real-world evidence from a European donor program, supporting current surgical practice that prioritizes split renal function and technical feasibility over arterial anatomy alone. Future multicenter and prospective studies—including perfusion imaging and more granular vascular characterization—are warranted to further refine donor selection and counseling.

5. Conclusions

In this retrospective cohort study, we found that living kidney donors left with a remnant kidney containing multiple renal arteries did not show statistically significant differences in long-term renal function or clinical outcomes compared to those left with a kidney with a single artery. No significant differences were observed in key parameters such as the eGFR, serum creatinine, incidence of hypertension, or metabolic and cardiovascular morbidity during long-term follow-up. Although certain postoperative complications were slightly more common in the MRA group, they were not associated with long-term sequelae or diminished renal function.

Our findings support the feasibility of retaining a kidney with multiple renal arteries in the donor when anatomical and functional criteria are otherwise met. These data may help inform surgical decision making and donor counseling in living kidney donation programs, though definitive conclusions about the impact of complex renal arterial anatomy on long-term donor outcomes are limited by the observational nature of the study.

Supplementary Materials: The following supporting information can be downloaded at https://www.mdpi.com/article/10.3390/jcm14176121/s1, Table S1: Multivariable Linear Regression Analysis of Factors Associated with eGFR at Last Follow-up; Table S2: Multivariable Logistic Regression Analysis of Factors Associated with Incident; Table S3: Post-hoc Power Analysis; Table S4: Power and Minimal Detectable Effects (MDE).

Author Contributions: Conceptualization, B.R. and J.S.; Methodology, T.K., J.S. and B.R.; Data curation, J.S., B.R., T.K., I.G., N.B., I.L., L.K., T.S., F.F., R.P., H.P., J.J.; Formal analysis, J.S. and B.R.; Writing—original draft preparation, T.K., B.R., and J.J.; Writing—review and editing, all authors; Supervision, B.R.; Project administration, B.R. All authors have read and agreed to the published version of the manuscript.

Funding: This research received no external funding.

Institutional Review Board Statement: This study has been conducted according to the Declaration of Helsinki; all organs were donated voluntarily with written informed consent, and this was conducted in accordance with the Declaration of Istanbul. The article is exempt from the local Ethical Committee approval (Institutional Review Board of Charité Hospital Berlin) because of this study's retrospective, noninterventional design and because patient data confidentiality and privacy were always maintained.

Informed Consent Statement: Informed consent for participation was obtained from all subjects involved in the study.

Data Availability Statement: The data presented in this study are available from the corresponding author upon reasonable request. Due to ethical considerations and institutional policies regarding donor privacy and data protection, individual-level clinical data cannot be made publicly available.

Conflicts of Interest: The authors declare no conflicts of interest.

Abbreviations

The following abbreviations are used in this manuscript:

MRAs	Multiple Renal Arteries
SRA	Single Renal Artery
eGFR	Estimated Glomerular Filtration Rate
CKD-EPI	Chronic Kidney Disease Epidemiology Collaboration
CT	Computed Tomography
MR	Magnetic Resonance
ESC	European Society of Cardiology
RRT	Renal Replacement Therapy
SD	Standard Deviation
IQR	Interquartile Range
BMI	Body Mass Index
ASA	American Society of Anesthesiologists
DM	Diabetes Mellitus
CVD	Cardiovascular Disease
HTN	Hypertension
SPSS	Statistical Package for the Social Sciences

References

1. Matas, A.J.; Schnitzler, M. Payment for living donor (vendor) kidneys: A cost-effectiveness analysis. *Am. J. Transplant.* **2004**, *4*, 216–221. [CrossRef]
2. Segev, D.L.; Muzaale, A.D.; Caffo, B.S.; Mehta, S.H.; Singer, A.L.; Taranto, S.E.; McBride, M.A.; Montgomery, R.A. Perioperative mortality and long-term survival following live kidney donation. *JAMA* **2010**, *303*, 959–966. [CrossRef]
3. Lentine, K.L.; Schnitzler, M.A.; Xiao, H.; Saab, G.; Salvalaggio, P.R.; Axelrod, D.; Davis, C.L.; Abbott, K.C.; Brennan, D.C. Racial variation in medical outcomes among living kidney donors. *N. Engl. J. Med.* **2010**, *363*, 724–732. [CrossRef] [PubMed]
4. Gürkan, A.; Kaçar, S.; Başak, K.; Varılsüha, C.; Karaca, C. Do multiple renal arteries restrict laparoscopic donor nephrectomy? *Transplant. Proc.* **2004**, *36*, 105–107. [CrossRef] [PubMed]
5. Lam, N.N.; Lentine, K.L.; Levey, A.S.; Kasiske, B.L.; Garg, A.X. Long-term medical risks to the living kidney donor. *Nat. Rev. Nephrol.* **2015**, *11*, 411–419. [CrossRef] [PubMed]
6. Carter, J.T.; Freise, C.E.; McTaggart, R.A.; Mahanty, H.D.; Kang, S.-M.; Chan, S.H.; Feng, S.; Roberts, J.P.; Posselt, A.M. Laparoscopic procurement of kidneys with multiple renal arteries is associated with increased ureteral complications in the recipient. *Am. J. Transplant.* **2005**, *5*, 1312–1318. [CrossRef]
7. Kok, N.F.M.; Dols, L.F.C.; Hunink, M.G.M.; Alwayn, I.P.J.; Tran, K.T.C.; Weimar, W.; Ijzermans, J.N.M. Complex Vascular Anatomy in Live Kidney Donation: Imaging and Conseque nces for Clinical Outcome. *Transplantation* **2008**, *85*, 1760–1765. [CrossRef]
8. Mahajan, A.D.; Patel, N.D.; Pal, L.S.; Bathe, S.; Darakh, P.P.; Patil, M. Retrospective Analysis of the Comparison Between Single Renal Artery V ersus Multiple Renal Arteries in Living Donor Kidney Transplant: Does It Affect the Outcome? *Exp. Clin. Transplant.* **2021**, *19*, 38–43. [CrossRef]
9. Ghazanfar, A.; Tavakoli, A.; Zaki, M.; Pararajasingam, R.; Campbell, T.; Parrott, N.; Augustine, T.; Riad, H. The Outcomes of Living Donor Renal Transplants With Multiple Renal Art eries: A Large Cohort Study With a Mean Follow-Up Period of 10 Years. *Transplant. Proc.* **2010**, *42*, 1654–1658. [CrossRef]
10. Marshall, A.G. Aberrant renal arteries and hypertension. *Lancet* **1951**, *2*, 701–705. [CrossRef]

11. Glodny, B.; Cromme, S.; Reimer, P.; Lennarz, M.; Winde, G.; Vetter, H. Hypertension associated with multiple renal arteries may be renin-depe ndent. *J. Hypertens.* **2000**, *18*, 1437–1444. [CrossRef]
12. Geyer, J.R. Incidence of Multiple Renal Arteries on Aortography. *JAMA* **1962**, *182*, 120. [CrossRef]
13. Bönner, G.; Dreesbach, H.; Helber, A.; Kaufmann, W. Hypertonus und multiple Nierenarterien. *DMW-Dtsch. Med. Wochenschr.* **1978**, *103*, 345–349. [CrossRef]
14. Nomura, G.; Kurosaki, M.; Kondo, T.; Takeuchi, J. Essential hypertension and multiple renal arteries. *Am. Heart J.* **1971**, *81*, 274–280. [CrossRef]
15. Gandhi, N.V.; Murad, D.N.; Nguyen, D.T.; Graviss, E.A.; Ibrahim, H.N. Hypertension and renal outcomes in normotensive kidney donors with mul tiple renal arteries. *Transpl. Int.* **2021**, *34*, 2382–2393. [CrossRef]
16. Levey, A.S.; Stevens, L.A.; Schmid, C.H.; Zhang, Y.L.; Castro, A.F., 3rd; Feldman, H.I.; Kusek, J.W.; Eggers, P.; Van Lente, F.; Greene, T.; et al. A new equation to estimate glomerular filtration rate. *Ann. Intern. Med.* **2009**, *150*, 604–612. [CrossRef]
17. Fehrman-Ekholm, I.; Möller, S.; Steinwall, J.; Nordén, G.; Lennerling, A.; Holmdahl, J.; Kvarnström, N.; Olausson, M. Single or Double Arteries in the Remnant Kidney After Donation: Influence on the Long-Term Outcome of the Donor. *Transplant. Proc.* **2009**, *41*, 764–765. [CrossRef] [PubMed]
18. Rizzari, M.D.; Suszynski, T.M.; Gillingham, K.J.; Matas, A.J.; Ibrahim, H.N. Outcome of living kidney donors left with multiple renal arteries. *Clin. Transplant.* **2012**, *26*, E7–E11. [CrossRef] [PubMed]
19. Choi, H.W.; Jung, J.W.; Jung, J.U.; Cho, H.J.; Hong, S.H.; Kim, J.C.; Park, Y.H.; Hwang, T.K. Feasibility and Safety of Performing Hand-assisted Laparoscopic Donor Nephrectomy for Patients with Multiple Renal Arteries. *Korean J. Urol.* **2008**, *49*, 443. [CrossRef]
20. Seet, C.; Clementoni, L.; Mohamed, I.; Khurram, M. O029 Long term outcomes of renal transplants in kidneys with multiple arteries. *Br. J. Surg.* **2022**, *109*, znac242-029. [CrossRef]
21. Afshari, A.T.; Fallah, M.; Alizadeh, M.; Makhdoomi, K.; Rahimi, E.; Vossoghian, S. Outcome of Kidney Transplantation From Living Donors With Multiple Renal Arteries Versus Single Renal Artery. *Iran. J. Kidney Dis.* **2016**, *10*, 85–90.
22. Şahin, S.; Özdemir, O.; Ekşi, M.; Evren, I.; Karadağ, S.; Arikan, Y.; Taşçı, A.İ. The effect of single or multiple arteries in the donor kidney on renal transplant surgical outcomes. *Ir. J. Med. Sci. (1971-)* **2022**, *192*, 929–934. [CrossRef]
23. Shabalin, A.I.; Rabkin, I.K.; Natsvlishvili, Z.G.; Germashev, V.G. Multiple renal arteries and renovascular hypertension. *Khirurgiia* **1989**, 24–29.
24. Benedetti, E.; Troppmann, C.; Gillingham, K.; Sutherland, D.E.R.; Payne, W.D.; Dunn, D.L.; Matas, A.J.; Najarian, J.S.; Gruessner, R.W.G. Short- and Long-Term Outcomes of Kidney Transplants with Multiple Renal Arteries. *Ann. Surg.* **1995**, *221*, 406. [CrossRef] [PubMed]
25. Ali-El-Dein, B.; Osman, Y.; Shokeir, A.A.; El-Dein, A.B.S.; Sheashaa, H.; Ghoneim, M.A. Multiple arteries in live donor renal transplantation: Surgical aspects and outcomes. *J. Urol.* **2003**, *169*, 2013–2017. [CrossRef] [PubMed]
26. Kek, H.Y.; Nicholas Wong, H.P.; Kyaw, L.; Lu, J.; Benjamin Goh, Y.S.; Tiong, H.Y. IP17-13 Dmsa-Based Pre-Donation Differential Renal Function Does Not Significantly Impact the New Baseline Glomerular Filtration Rate: A Retrospective Five-Year Cohort Study of 124 Kidney Donors. *J. Urol.* **2025**, *213*, e888. [CrossRef]
27. Jo, E.-A.; Lee, J.; Moon, S.; Kim, J.S.; Han, A.; Ha, J.; Kim, Y.C.; Min, S. The role of artificial intelligence measured preoperative kidney volume in predicting kidney function loss in elderly kidney donors: A multicenter cohort study. *Int. J. Surg.* **2024**, *110*, 7169–7176. [CrossRef]
28. Fananapazir, G.; Benzl, R.; Corwin, M.T.; Chen, L.-X.; Sageshima, J.; Stewart, S.L.; Troppmann, C. Predonation Volume of Future Remnant Cortical Kidney Helps Predict Postdonation Renal Function in Live Kidney Donors. *Radiology* **2018**, *288*, 153–157. [CrossRef]
29. Rivas-Nieto, A.C.; Cárcamo, C.P.; Munarriz, C.L.; Miyahira, J. Early physiological and morphological changes in the remnant kidney of living donors. *Rev. Peru. Med. Exp. Y Salud Publica* **2020**, *37*, 733–738. [CrossRef]

Journal of
Clinical Medicine

MDPI

Review

Recurrence of Glomerular Diseases (GN) After Kidney Transplantation: A Narrative Review

Abbal Koirala, Aditi Singh and Duvuru Geetha *

Division of Nephrology, Johns Hopkins School of Medicine, 5501 Hopkins Bayview Circle, Floor 1, Baltimore, MD 21224, USA; akoiral1@jh.edu (A.K.); asing148@jh.edu (A.S.)
* Correspondence: dgeetha1@jhmi.edu

Abstract: Recurrence of the original glomerular disease (GN) poses a significant threat to kidney transplant function and longevity. The probability and severity of this recurrence vary, with C3 glomerulopathy and certain forms of FSGS exhibiting particularly high rates. Kidney transplant GN recurrence risk hinges on the characteristics of the initial GN, recipient/donor genetics, recipient age, donor type, end-stage kidney disease (ESRD) progression rate, and proteinuria levels. Standard immunosuppression has limited efficacy in preventing primary disease recurrence; however, agent selection and induction therapy can influence the risk for specific GNs. Diagnosing recurrent GN involves a comprehensive approach, including clinical evaluation, laboratory tests (such as proteinuria, hematuria, and specific biomarkers like anti-PLA2R for membranous nephropathy or complement for C3G), and, critically, an allograft biopsy analyzed with light, immunofluorescence, and electron microscopy. Treatment strategies are evolving towards targeted therapies, such as rituximab for antibody-mediated GN and complement inhibitors for C3G, moving away from broad immunosuppression. This narrative literature review provides practical monitoring algorithms for post-transplant settings, synthesizing information on the incidence, predictors, diagnostic strategies, and therapeutic options for various glomerular disease subtypes. The methodology involved searching MEDLINE, Embase, and Cochrane databases from 1996 to 2025, prioritizing systematic reviews, cohort studies, registries, and interventional reports. Eligibility criteria included adult transplant recipients and English-language reports on recurrent glomerular disease outcomes, excluding most single-patient case reports. Limitations include potential selection bias, omission of relevant studies, and the absence of a formal risk-of-bias assessment or meta-analysis. The evidence base is heterogeneous, with inconsistent outcome reporting and scarce randomized controlled trials. Future efforts should focus on developing predictive biomarkers, standardizing diagnostic and response criteria, conducting multicenter prospective cohorts and pragmatic trials, and creating shared registries with harmonized data.

Keywords: glomerular disease (GN); IgA nephropathy (IgAN); focal segmental glomerulosclerosis (FSGS); membranoproliferative glomerulonephritis (MPGN); C3 glomerulopathy (C3G); membranous nephropathy (MN); recurrent lupus nephritis (RLN); anti-glomerular basement membrane disease (anti-GBM disease); ANCA-associated vasculitis (AAV)

1. Introduction

Glomerular diseases (GN) are a leading global cause of end-stage renal disease (ESRD). In the United States, GN accounts for 7% of new dialysis patients and 13% of kidney transplant recipients, underscoring its substantial global impact on chronic kidney disease [1].

Despite the considerable benefits of kidney transplantation, the long-term survival of the transplanted allograft is seriously and continuously threatened by the recurrence of the original GN or the development of de novo GN. This recurrence is a key contributor to early allograft failure, ranking as the third leading cause of graft loss within ten years after renal transplantation [1–5]. GN recurrence post-transplant varies from 3 to 15% generally [1], but certain types, like dense deposit disease, can reach 100% [2]. Common GNs (IgA nephropathy, focal and segmental glomerulosclerosis, membranous nephropathy) also show notable recurrence, although usually lower than 100%. This variability underscores the importance of early detection and management to improve long-term outcomes for kidney transplant recipients with GN.

The timing of recurrence varies. While risk increases with time, some GNs, such as focal and segmental glomerulosclerosis (FSGS) and C3 glomerulopathy (C3G), can recur within days or weeks. This bimodal pattern suggests different mechanisms: early recurrence due to active, persistent systemic factors (e.g., permeability factors, antinephrin antibodies in FSGS, complement dysregulation in C3G); later recurrence due to gradual reestablishment of the original disease process, possibly influenced by the allograft environment or long-term interactions with the immunosuppressive regimen.

The recognition of recurrent GN as a major risk to long-term graft survival represents a shift in post-transplant care. While preventing and treating acute rejection remains vital, managing disease recurrence is now equally crucial for durable allograft function in patients transplanted for GN. This necessitates a deeper understanding of recurrence factors for each specific GN and the development of targeted preventive and therapeutic strategies.

A fundamental challenge is the ongoing presence of the underlying systemic disease, which is not cured by transplantation. The transplanted kidney is susceptible to the same disease processes that damaged the original kidneys. This vulnerability requires rigorous patient care, including a thorough pre-transplant risk assessment to identify individuals at higher recurrence risk, as well as aggressive, individualized post-transplant monitoring and management. Understanding that transplantation addresses organ failure but not necessarily the systemic disease is vital for optimizing long-term outcomes for transplant recipients.

2. Methods

This narrative literature review aims to provide practical monitoring algorithms for the post-transplant setting. It synthesizes information regarding the incidence, predictors, diagnostic strategies, and therapeutic options for various glomerular disease subtypes. The review's methodology involved searching MEDLINE, Embase, and Cochrane databases for publications from 1996 to 2025. The search utilized controlled vocabulary and keywords related to glomerulonephritis, recurrence, and kidney transplantation. Priority was given to systematic reviews, cohort studies, registries, and interventional reports, with findings narratively synthesized by disease entity, emphasizing clinical applicability. Eligibility criteria included adult transplant recipients and reports containing data on the incidence, predictors, diagnosis, treatment, or outcomes of recurrent glomerular disease. Only English-language reports were included, and single-patient case reports were excluded unless uniquely informative. However, this review has several limitations, including potential selection bias, possible omission of relevant studies, and the absence of a formal risk-of-bias assessment or meta-analysis. The evidence base is heterogeneous, with variability in diagnostic criteria and outcome definitions. Most data are derived from retrospective cohorts and transplant registries, which are subject to indication and survivorship biases. Outcome reporting is inconsistent, and response criteria are not standardized. Randomized controlled trials in kidney transplant recipients are scarce, and generalizability from native kidney disease studies is uncertain. The strength of evidence was qualitatively graded as high, moderate, or low, considering study design, sample size, consistency, and directness.

Future initiatives should prioritize the development and validation of predictive biomarkers for recurrence risk stratification. Additionally, efforts should focus on establishing standardized diagnostic and response criteria specifically adapted for the transplant setting. Conducting multicenter prospective cohort studies and pragmatic trials, alongside the creation of shared registries with harmonized data elements, are also crucial next steps.

2.1. General Epidemiology and Impact of Recurrent GN

2.1.1. Overall Prevalence of GN Recurrence Post-Transplant

The recurrence of GN after kidney transplantation is observed in 3% to 15% of cases. However, this prevalence is probably underestimated for several reasons. Selection bias in patient listing for transplantation is a major factor, as systematic variations in the selection and listing of ESRD patients with different GN subtypes and observation period can distort reported incidences.

Another critical factor is the inconsistency in biopsy practices across transplant centers. Centers that regularly perform "protocol" biopsies (scheduled biopsies regardless of symptoms) report higher recurrence rates than those that only perform "for-cause" biopsies (biopsies performed due to clinical signs of dysfunction). This suggests that many recurrences may be subclinical and only identifiable through routine histological examination. Furthermore, the diagnosis of recurrent GN may require electron microscopy, which is not routinely performed. Additionally, difficulties in accurately determining the primary GN diagnosis in the native kidney can also lead to underestimation.

Recurrent glomerular disease increases in prevalence over time, becoming the second leading histopathological diagnosis after antibody-mediated rejection at 10 years post-transplant. The risk of recurrence is generally proportional to time since transplantation, with most allograft failures occurring within 3–5 years of recurrence. However, C3G and FSGS can recur earlier, sometimes within months. This temporal variability highlights the need for tailored monitoring strategies tailored to the specific GN subtype.

2.1.2. Impact of Recurrence on Allograft Survival and Patient Outcomes

Recurrent GN is a substantial contributor to premature allograft failure, representing a critical challenge in the long-term success of kidney transplantation. Patients who experience recurrent GN are twice as likely to lose their allograft compared to those who do not, with approximately 45% of affected grafts failing within 5 years of recurrence [3,6–8]. This profound impact on graft longevity positions recurrent disease as the third most common cause of graft failure 10 years after renal transplantation, following death with a functioning graft and chronic rejection.

The severity of the impact of recurrence on graft survival varies considerably depending on the specific GN subtype. For instance, IgA Nephropathy (IgAN) is generally associated with better long-term allograft and patient outcomes compared to other GN subtypes, even after recurrence. In contrast, MPGN (membranoproliferative glomerulonephritis), particularly dense deposit disease (DDD), is associated with a substantially poorer allograft survival rate following recurrence. FSGS also presents a high risk of allograft failure upon recurrence, with rates as high as 50%. This differential impact highlights that while recurrence is a broad concern, its specific consequences are highly dependent on the underlying disease pathology.

The clinical implications of these observations are significant. The high rate of graft loss associated with recurrence means that patients with certain GN types face an ongoing battle even after receiving a new kidney. This situation creates a complex dynamic where the initial success of transplantation must be continuously protected against the re-emergence of the original disease. The variability in outcomes across different GN subtypes suggests that a "one-size-fits-all" approach to post-transplant management is insufficient. Instead, management strategies must be precisely adapted to each GN type's specific characteristics and recurrence risks. This tailored approach is crucial for maintaining graft function and enhancing the overall quality of life and long-term survival for transplant recipients.

Key points are as follows:

- Recurrence of glomerular diseases (GN) after kidney transplantation is a significant factor in long-term graft loss, with varying rates depending on the specific GN subtype.
- Diagnosis relies on clinical suspicion (proteinuria, hematuria, declining graft function) and allograft biopsy, with protocol biopsies revealing more subclinical cases than "for-cause" biopsies.
- Management and monitoring strategies for recurrent GN are highly individualized based on the specific disease subtype, requiring a comprehensive understanding of each GN's immunopathogenesis and risk factors.

2.2. Specific GN Subtypes and Their Recurrence Characteristics (See Figure 1 and Tables 1–4)

2.2.1. IgA Nephropathy (IgAN)

IgA nephropathy (IgAN) is the most common primary GN. It leads to ESRD in 15–20% of patients within 10 years, and 20–40% within 20 years of diagnosis.

Prevalence and Time to Recurrence: IgAN recurrence after kidney transplant is common, with histological recurrence rates of up to 51% at 5 years. Clinical recurrence often appears after 5 years. Rates vary from 10% to 30% in "for-cause" biopsy studies and from 25% to 53% in "protocol" biopsy studies, indicating that many subclinical cases are detected only through systematic histological examination [9–12]. The median recurrence time is approximately 59 months (range, 16–90 months).

Graft Outcome: Recurrent IgAN is common, negatively impacting graft survival and leading to allograft loss in up to 40% of patients (60% due to recurrence). This significantly lowers 10-year graft survival, with a 5-year allograft failure rate of 42%. While recurrent IgAN is common, its long-term impact on allograft and patient outcomes is generally considered better compared to other GN subtypes [5,9,10,13,14].

Risk Factors:

- Recipient Factors: Younger age at IgAN diagnosis and at transplant [9,15], faster progression from IgAN to ESRD [15,16], pre-transplant tonsillectomy, prior kidney transplantation (43% increased risk), hemodialysis as KRT [15], and preemptive transplantation [9].
- Immunosuppression and Induction Therapy: Higher recurrence rates are associated with steroid-avoidance/early steroid withdrawal and no induction therapy. ATG induction, mycophenolate mofetil, anti-IL-2R antibody induction, and pre-transplant tonsillectomy may decrease recurrence. Post-transplant mTOR inhibitors increase recurrence risk [15,17].
- Immunological Factors: Pre- and post-transplant donor-specific antibodies (DSAs) significantly increase recurrence risk (HR 2.74 and 6.65, respectively [9]). Other risk factors include the presence of Gd-IgA1, IgG anti-Gd-IgA1, glycan-specific IgG antibodies, and soluble CD89 [18], as well as sIgA levels post-transplantation [19].
- Genetic Factors: IgAN is a genetically diverse polygenic disease involving MHC (HLA) and non-MHC susceptibility alleles. Lower HLA/HLA-DR mismatches and living donors are associated with higher recurrence rates [15].

- Clinical Course: Crescentic IgAN, an aggressive pre-transplant condition, increases the risk of early, aggressive recurrence. Recurrence is associated with higher proteinuria in the initial year post-transplant and a more rapid eGFR decline [20].

Histology: Histologically, recurrent IgAN is defined by dominant or co-dominant IgA mesangial staining on immunofluorescence, often accompanied by mesangial expansion and hypercellularity on light microscopy.

Immunological and Pathological Mechanisms: IgAN recurrence is a complex process involving the continued production and deposition of abnormal IgA1 (Gd-IgA1) and immune complexes in the mesangium of the transplanted kidney. IgG anti-Gd-IgA1 and glycan-specific IgG antibodies contribute to this. The "multi-hit hypothesis" highlights genetic and environmental interplay in the pathogenesis. Post-transplant DSAs increase risk, suggesting an alloimmune component that exacerbates the autoimmune process. Histologically, recurrent IgAN shows IgA deposition, mesangial hypercellularity, and segmental glomerulosclerosis in allograft biopsies [21,22].

Treatment of Recurrent IgAN Post-Transplantation

No standardized treatment exists for recurrent IgA nephropathy (IgAN) following kidney transplantation. Management primarily involves supportive care, with renin–angiotensin system (RAS) inhibitors (ACE inhibitors or ARBs) recommended to reduce proteinuria and protect kidney function [10].

For active or severe recurrence, a regimen of intravenous methylprednisolone (500 mg daily for three days at months 1, 3, and 5) combined with oral prednisone (0.5 mg/kg every other day for six months) may be considered [23]. However, more extensive randomized controlled studies are needed to establish a gold standard treatment.

In severe or treatment-resistant cases, particularly those with endocapillary proliferation or crescentic lesions, additional therapies like cyclophosphamide [24–26], rituximab [27,28], and, rarely, complement inhibitors such as eculizumab [29], have shown potential in limited studies and individual reports.

Tonsillectomy one year post-transplant has been linked to reduced histological IgAN recurrence (11.1% vs. 55.6%), decreased serum Gd-IgA1 levels, and reduced mesangial IgA and Gd-IgA1 immunoreactivity compared to controls [30]. Modifications to maintenance immunosuppression regimens, such as using everolimus with tacrolimus and corticosteroids versus MMF-based regimens with tacrolimus and corticosteroids, have shown a correlation with reduced recurrence in specific scenarios; however, further research is required to confirm their efficacy [31]. Dual BAFF-APRIL inhibitors [32,33], including Atacicept and Povitacicept, which are currently being investigated for treating native IgAN to reduce Gd-IgA1 immune complex production, may prove beneficial in preventing IgAN recurrence after kidney transplantation.

Screening and monitoring: Microhematuria and proteinuria screening: monthly for the first month, quarterly for the first year, then annually. Emerging biomarkers (IgA, IgA-IgG complexes, Gd-IgA1, anti-Gd-IgA1 autoantibodies) are investigational. New or worsening hematuria, proteinuria, or graft dysfunction necessitates allograft biopsy to confirm recurrence and exclude other causes [10,16].

2.2.2. Focal Segmental Glomerulosclerosis (FSGS)

FSGS is the most frequent glomerular disease causing ESRD globally, posing a challenge in kidney transplantation due to high recurrence. It is a non-specific histological finding of various podocytopathies, and differentiating types is crucial for post-transplant care, as primary FSGS often recurs, unlike other forms [34,35].

Prevalence and Time to Recurrence: Recurrent FSGS (rFSGS) is a severe complication following kidney transplantation, with reported incidence rates ranging from 17% to 55% [36]. The recurrence rate in first kidney grafts for primary FSGS is estimated at 40–60%, and this can rise to over 80% in patients whose initial graft failed due to recurrent FSGS [37]. Typically, recurrence manifests early in the post-transplant period, with a median onset of 1.5 months. It can be aggressive, leading to nephrotic-range proteinuria within hours to days after transplantation. Most recurrences are observed within the first two years following kidney transplantation [36,37].

Graft Outcome: rFSGS frequently causes premature allograft failure, with a 5-year graft survival rate of 52% compared to 83% in non-recurrent cases [36]. Half of the patients experiencing recurrence lose their graft within 5 years, with most graft losses occurring within the first 2 years after disease recurrence. De novo FSGS shows slower progression and better long-term survival (60% vs. 33.3% probability of graft survival) than recurrent FSGS [38].

Risk Factors:

- Recipient Factors: rFSGS is highly influenced by prior allograft recurrence (80% risk). Other factors include younger age at onset, rapid ESRD progression, BMI at transplantation, and nephrotic syndrome with low serum albumin (<2.5 g/L) at diagnosis [39,40]. Pre-transplant antinephrin antibodies predict FSGS recurrence, showing high specificity [41,42]. In recurrence cases, allograft biopsies reveal co-localized glomerular deposition of nephrin and IgG, suggesting a pathogenic role needing further investigation [41].
- Genetic Factors: Familial FSGS, due to podocyte slit diaphragm protein mutations (excluding podocin), generally has low or no recurrence risk [43,44]. Pre-transplant genetic testing is crucial for risk assessment, identifying suitable living donors, and avoiding unnecessary immunosuppression.
- Histological Features: The native kidney's FSGS subtype (e.g., collapsing, tip lesions) does not significantly impact recurrence risk or type of FSGS seen in the allograft [45].
- Donor Factors: rFSGS and donor type are debated. Some studies weakly link living donors to higher recurrence [40] while others find no independent association. Despite this, living donor kidney transplantation generally results in improved graft survival.

Immunological and Pathological Mechanisms: rFSGS is linked to circulating permeability factors like Soluble Urokinase-Type Plasminogen Activator Receptor (suPAR), Cardiotrophin-like Cytokine Factor 1 (CLCF-1), plasminogen activator inhibitor type-1 (PAI-1), and angiotensin II type 1 receptors (AT1Rs) [46]. This is supported by observations of recurrence despite immunosuppression, maternal–child transmission, and the effectiveness of plasmapheresis in reducing proteinuria and preventing recurrence [47]. Experimental evidence shows that FSGS patient serum induces proteinuria in rats [48,49] and affects podocytes in cell cultures [50].

Antinephrin antibodies are implicated in primary podocytopathies, found in 44% of adults with minimal change disease (MCD) and 9% with pFSGS in one study [51]. A link between antinephrin antibodies and disease activity was observed, hinting at a possible pathogenic function, though further investigation is needed. Another study identified them in 45% of MCD and 37.5% of pFSGS patients [52]. Furthermore, the presence of pre-transplant antinephrin antibodies has recently been linked to rFSGS.

Histology: The only initial finding in allograft biopsies for recurrent FSGS may be diffuse podocyte foot process effacement on electron microscopy, alongside new-onset progressive proteinuria.

Recurrence Prevention

Evidence regarding post-transplant recurrence prevention strategies is both limited and contradictory. KDIGO 2020 guidelines advise against routine pre-transplant plasma exchange (PLEX) or rituximab (RTX) to lower the risk of rFSGS (2D) [37,53]. Although previous studies found no significant effect of prophylactic PLEX on rFSGS, these studies were limited by small sample sizes, retrospective analyses, and lack of randomization [54]. Conversely, a recent retrospective study indicated that pre-transplant PLEX was associated with a reduced rFSGS (34.8% recurrence risk without PLEX vs. 9.4% with PLEX) [55]. Similarly, data on prophylactic RTX use are limited. A meta-analysis suggests that RTX, either alone or with PLEX, or PLEX alone, does not substantially decrease the risk of rFSGS [56].

Recurrence Management of Post-Transplant FSGS

Treatment options for rFSGS are limited and have not changed much. Daily proteinuria monitoring post-transplant is vital for early recurrence detection. Rituximab (RTX) and plasma exchange (PLEX) are common initial treatments for pFSGS recurrence (80% of cases). RTX acts on podocytes and depletes B cells, reducing permeability factors and antinephrin antibodies. PLEX removes circulating pathogenic factors. Early RTX response is attributed to its direct podocyte-stabilizing effect through SMPDL3b [57].

Immunoadsorption selectively removes immunoglobulins, preserving coagulation factors, unlike plasma exchange (PLEX), but is more expensive and less available, with no proven clinical superiority [58,59]. The TANGO study of 61 rFSGS patients treated with PLEX ± rituximab (RTX) showed 21% complete remission, 36% partial remission, and 43% no response [39]. A French study by Lanaret et al. [60] comparing standard care (PLEX, CNI, steroids) with or without RTX reported 46.6% complete and 33.1% partial remission rates, with significantly better 10-year graft survival in responders (64.7%) versus nonresponders (17.9%). For plasma exchange (PLEX) or rituximab (RTX)-unresponsive cases, alternative strategies, targeting specific mechanisms in podocytes are suggested, including ACTH gel [61,62], LDL pheresis [63–65], abatacept, and ofatumumab [66,67].

Screening and monitoring of rFSGS: For potential early, fulminant FSGS recurrence, high-risk patients need more frequent post-transplant proteinuria screening: daily for week 1, weekly for 4 weeks, then quarterly for a year, and annually thereafter. Close monitoring, allograft biopsy for confirmation, and prompt, intensive treatment are crucial [10,16]. Pre-transplant genetic testing is essential to rule out genetic causes of FSGS, which have a low likelihood of recurrence. Biomarkers like suPAR, CLC-1, AT1R-Ab, anti-CD40, IL-13, and antinephrin antibodies are being explored.

2.2.3. Membranous Nephropathy (MN)

Membranous Nephropathy (MN), a major cause of kidney failure and nephrotic syndrome in adults, recurs post-transplant (10–45%, 31% cumulative incidence at 10 years). Recurrence averages 6.3 years, longer than other glomerular diseases. Early recurrence (6–12 months) implies the presence of pre-existing antibodies, while late onset (around 5 years) suggests new antibody production.

De novo MN, rare in transplanted kidneys, is PLA2R-negative and presents with proteinuria, leading to poorer outcomes than recurrent MN (which is PLA2R-positive). Often linked to alloimmune responses and anti-HLA antibodies, it may show concurrent antibody-mediated rejection histologically and lacks IgG4 dominance, differentiating it from primary MN. Its clinical course is more aggressive, with a higher risk of allograft loss [68,69].

Graft Outcome: While most studies on recurrent membranous nephropathy (MN) indicate no significant independent link with graft loss [70,71], de novo MN might carry a more severe prognosis for graft survival in certain situations. The reported graft failure rate for de novo MN is 11.7 per 100 person-years, markedly higher than the 3.7 per 100 person-years observed in recurrent MN [68].

Risk Factors:

- Immunological Factors: Elevated pre-transplant anti-PLA2R antibodies are the primary risk factor for recurrence, with a 70% risk in positive patients vs. 30% in negative [7,37,71–73]. High pre-transplant PLA2R levels and post-transplant persistence/reappearance indicate earlier and more aggressive disease.
- Recipient Factors: Higher MN post-transplant recurrence is linked to female sex, younger age [5], recipient HLA-A3 antigen [68], high pre-transplant proteinuria [72], and faster ESRD progression [71].
- Genetic Factors: Donor HLA-D and PLA2R1 risk alleles can increase MN recurrence [74,75].
- Donor Factors: Older studies suggest a higher recurrence rate in living- vs. deceased-donor transplants, especially living-related, implying a genetic link [68].

Immunological and Pathological Mechanisms: Recurrent membranous nephropathy (MN) is mainly caused by recipient anti-PLA2R IgG4 autoantibodies binding to donor kidney podocyte antigens like the M-type phospholipase A2 receptor (PLA2R). These antibodies, found in 70–80% of primary MN patients, are key to immune complex formation in recurrent MN, which then activate complement and lead to subepithelial immune deposit formation, podocyte injury, and proteinuria [76]. Anti-PLA2R antibody identification aids MN risk assessment, though new antigens still affect recurrence rates.

Histology: Recurrent MN is histologically characterized by subepithelial immune complex formation, granular IgG, and less frequent complement deposition along the glomerular basement membrane, and detectable PLA2R antigen in immune deposits. It may present subclinically, often detected on protocol biopsies before overt proteinuria [72,77].

Treatment of Post-Transplant Recurrent MN

Post-transplant recurrent membranous nephropathy is initially managed by optimizing conservative, antiproteinuric measures (ACE inhibitors/ARBs, strict adherence to the existing immunosuppressant regimen). Rituximab is the favored initial immunosuppressive therapy for proteinuria >1 g/day, showing better remission rates than conservative management [71,72,78]. Monitoring anti-PLA2R antibody levels post-transplantation is crucial for detecting recurrence, potentially requiring biopsy and more intensive treatment [78]. Regular antibody measurements are advised for PLA2R-associated disease for 6–12 months post-transplant. Biopsy should be considered if proteinuria is 0.3–1.0 g/day and antibody levels are rising or high [71,78].

NKF and KDIGO guidelines emphasize tailored treatment for refractory or relapsing disease, though rituximab is preferred when additional immunosuppression is required. Case reports and small series suggest obinutuzumab as a promising alternative to rituximab for post-transplant MN recurrence when rituximab is ineffective [79–81].

Screening and monitoring of recurrent MN: KDIGO guidelines suggest monthly proteinuria checks for 6–12 months post-transplant to screen for recurrent membranous nephropathy. For PLA2R disease, monitor anti-PLA2R antibodies monthly (high titers) to quarterly (undetectable) based on pre-transplant levels. Biopsy if proteinuria exceeds 1 g/day. Consider biopsy for rising/high anti-PLA2R titers even with proteinuria in the 0.3–1.0 g/day range, indicating early recurrence. For non-PLA2R MN, only proteinuria monitoring is recommended, with biopsy if it exceeds 1 g/day [78].

2.2.4. Membranoproliferative Glomerulonephritis (MPGN)/C3 Glomerulopathy (C3G)

MPGN is classified as immune complex GN (ICGN) or complement-mediated GN, also known as C3 glomerulopathy (C3G), a rare, progressive kidney disease caused by dysregulation of the alternative complement pathway.

Prevalence and Time to Recurrence: MPGN recurrence post-transplant is 20–45%, higher in complement-mediated forms (C3G) and with monoclonal gammopathy (IC-MPGN). Polyclonal immune complex-mediated MPGN has a lower risk, while C3G recurrence can exceed 60–70%. DDD, a C3G subtype (formerly MPGN type II), has a near 100% late recurrence rate. C3G recurs early after transplant [37,82,83]. The median time to recurrence for C3G ranges from 1.1 to 28 months, with some recurrences as early as 9 days post-transplant [84].

Graft Outcome: MPGN recurrence, especially C3G, negatively impacts graft survival, which is poorer than other GN subtypes. Half of recurrent MPGN patients may lose allografts. C3G recurrence leads to graft failure in 11–77% (mostly >50%) [82–86]. Graft loss is more common and sooner in DDD than in C3 glomerulonephritis [84].

Risk Factors for IC-MPGN

- Recipient Factors: Lower BMI at transplant, crescents in original biopsy, more glomeruli with crescents in native biopsy [10,85], shorter dialysis duration before kidney transplantation [87], and prior graft loss from MPGN [10] are all factors.
- Immunological Factors: Lower serum complement and monoclonal gammopathy [1,53,82] correlate with higher recurrence and poorer outcomes. Recurrence is less common in polyclonal IC-MPGN, especially if the underlying cause is controlled [83].
- Donor Factors: Higher recurrence rates of ICGN have been linked to living-related allografts and preemptive transplantation [82].

Risk Factors for C3G

- Recipient Factors: Young age at diagnosis, an aggressive course of native kidney disease, male sex, and pre-emptive transplantation are risk factors [53,84]. Some studies have noted low complements as risk factors at the time of transplantation [53]. Paraproteinemia-associated C3G can drive complement dysregulation and is associated with more aggressive and earlier recurrence [88].
- Delayed graft function, ischemia–reperfusion injury, and post-transplant infection can activate the complement system, potentially leading to early recurrence, especially in patients with complement dysregulation [88].
- Immunological Factors: Genetic or acquired alternative complement pathway abnormalities (e.g., factor H or I mutations, C3NeFs) are linked to a high risk of C3G recurrence after transplant, but the specific predictive value of genetic versus acquired causes is not fully defined per KDIGO guidelines [53,84,89,90].
- Donor Factors: While some reports suggest increased C3G recurrence with living donors, this is not consistently replicated [84].

Immunological and Pathological Mechanisms: MPGN/C3G recurrence post-transplant stems from unaddressed complement dysregulation, leading to uncontrolled alternative complement pathway (ACP) activation. This dysregulation can be inherited (e.g., *CFHR5*, *CFHR3-1* mutations) or acquired (e.g., autoantibodies like C3 nephritic factor, anti-CFH antibodies, or monoclonal immunoglobulins inhibiting complement regulatory proteins or acting as C3NeF). Ischemia–reperfusion injury and post-transplant infections can also trigger ACP. Histologically, recurrence shows mesangial hypercellularity, endocapillary proliferation, MPGN patterns, or crescentic GN with dominant C3 deposition on immunofluorescence (intensity $\geq$ 2+) [88,91]. Electron microscopy reveals characteristic dense deposits (in DDD) or electron-dense deposits in subendothelial, mesangial, or subepithelial spaces.

Treatment of IC-MPGN Recurrence Post-Kidney Transplantation

Underlying causes (e.g., hepatitis C, infections, dysproteinemia, malignancy) of IC-MPGN should be ruled out and treated. Idiopathic cases require individualized therapy due to limited data and varied outcomes.

Glucocorticoids are initial immunosuppressants. Alternatives like mycophenolate mofetil, rituximab [92,93], or cyclophosphamide [94] are used if there are contraindications, intolerance, or inadequate response. KDOQI and KDIGO guidelines support this, emphasizing individualized therapy based on patient risk and comorbidities [92,95]. There is emerging data with pegcetacoplan in IC-MPGN and C3G, as stated below.

Treatment of C3G Recurrence Post-Kidney Transplantation

RAAS blockers and lipid-lowering agents are used as supportive treatment. Standard immunosuppressants often fail to prevent C3G recurrence and progression [88]. For C3G recurrence, targeting complement inhibition is crucial. Eculizumab (C5 antibody) for recurring C3G and DDD yields variable results, with some patients showing improved graft function and reduced proteinuria, and others showing no response. This is likely due to diverse complement pathway dysregulation. It is most effective in terminal pathway activation, but consistent patient response is not guaranteed [88–91,96].

Iptacopan, a factor B inhibitor, shows promise for post-transplant C3G recurrence, improving clinical, lab, and histological markers [97]. Early studies of pegcetacoplan, a C3 inhibitor for C3G (including post-transplant recurrent DDD), show promise in pediatric patients with native kidney C3G [98,99]. These studies indicate it can reduce proteinuria, raise C3 levels, and stabilize or improve kidney function with good short-term safety. The Phase 2 NOBLE study (NCT04572854) demonstrated that pegcetacoplan reduced C3c staining and proteinuria, stabilized eGFR, and improved complement biomarkers in kidney transplant recipients with recurrent C3G or IC-MPGN, compared to the standard of care [100]. VALIANT study (NCT05067127) showed positive results in IC-MPGN/C3G, reducing proteinuria and C3c staining, and stabilizing kidney function. The KDOQI commentary on the 2021 KDIGO guideline emphasizes the need for clinical trial enrollment for C3G due to limited evidence and the potential for personalized complement-targeted treatments.

Screening and monitoring of MPGN/C3G recurrence: Recurrent MPGN or C3G involves close clinical and lab monitoring, including serial creatinine/eGFR, regular proteinuria/hematuria checks, and periodic complement level assessments (C3, C4) with monoclonal protein screening. Protocol (surveillance) kidney biopsies are highly recommended, especially in the first 1–2 years, as early recurrence is often subclinical [101,102]. Prompt biopsies are crucial for unexplained graft dysfunction, new or worsening proteinuria, or hematuria. Complement biomarker profiling and genetic testing are considered in select cases to guide prognosis and therapy. Despite these guidelines, no standardized protocol exists; monitoring is individualized based on risk factors, disease subtype, and evolving evidence [37,88,103].

2.2.5. Anti-Glomerular Basement Membrane (Anti-GBM) Disease

Prevalence and Time to Recurrence: Anti-GBM disease recurrence post-transplant is rare (1.9–4%), attributed to its monophasic nature and sustained immunosuppression [104]. One study found only one recurrence in 53 patients, occurring 5 years post-transplant [104].

Graft Outcome: Anti-GBM disease recurrence is rare but strongly linked to graft loss, often causing rapid, irreversible failure within weeks to months. Due to this low recurrence, long-term patient and graft survival post-transplant are excellent, comparable to other immune-mediated diseases.

Risk Factors:

- Immunological Factors: Circulating anti-GBM antibodies at transplant are a key risk factor for graft loss due to recurrence [104]. KDIGO guidelines advise delaying transplantation until antibodies are undetectable for at least 6 months [10,95].
- Immunosuppression: Cessation or reduction of immunosuppressive drugs is a significant risk factor for reactivation [104]. Patients on low-dose or no immunosuppression are at higher risk.
- Other Factors: Other potential risk factors, such as the pre-transplant disease course, time from initial disease to transplantation, or donor type, have not been shown to predict recurrence [10,85].

Atypical anti-GBM, characterized by linear GBM staining for monotypic or polytypic Ig without a diffuse crescentic pattern, is common post-transplant. A case series of 6 patients found that recurrence averaged 3.8 months post-transplant. All had monotypic Ig staining, negative serum anti-GBM antibodies, and negative serum monoclonal disease and experienced benign courses with no graft loss. Most were on maintenance immunosuppression with good outcomes; 3 received plasma cell therapies due to identifiable clones [105].

De novo anti-GBM disease, a rare complication (2–3% of cases) of post-transplant Alport disease, stems from an alloimmune response to neoantigens within the allograft. Although maintenance immunosuppression can mitigate glomerular involvement, the presence of this disease leads to rapid graft loss. Subsequent transplants may result in more aggressive disease [95].

Immunological and pathological mechanisms:

Recurrence of anti-GBM disease post-kidney transplant is caused by the re-emergence of anti-GBM antibodies that target the non-collagenous domain of the $\alpha3$ chain of type IV collagen within the glomerular basement membrane. The precise immunological mechanisms driving recurrence are not fully understood, but potential triggers include the cessation or reduction of immunosuppression, which can reactivate anti-GBM antibodies. Additionally, cellular rejection may expose previously hidden epitopes, thereby inducing the formation of antibodies against them. The existence of antibody-negative cases highlights the limitations of relying solely on serological monitoring [106,107].

The highest risk of recurrence is observed in patients with detectable circulating anti-GBM antibodies at the time of transplant. While recurrence is uncommon when transplantation occurs during serological quiescence, if it does happen, it leads to rapid and severe allograft injury, often manifesting as crescentic glomerulonephritis. Immunopathology typically reveals linear IgG deposition along the GBM, complement activation, and inflammatory cell recruitment.

Treatment of recurrent anti-GBM disease:

Recurrent post-transplant anti-GBM disease needs immediate treatment: high-dose corticosteroids (e.g., IV methylprednisolone 500–1000 mg daily for 3 days, then oral prednisone 1 mg/kg/day, tapered clinically), daily/QOD plasma exchange until anti-GBM antibodies are undetectable, and cyclophosphamide (oral or IV, adjusted by kidney function and cytopenias). Refractory cases may use rituximab or immunoadsorption, as per KDIGO guidelines and case series [16,78,95,106]. Once antibodies are undetectable, maintenance immunosuppression beyond standard post-transplant care is usually unnecessary.

Screening and monitoring of anti-GBM recurrence: Post-transplant, it is recommended to screen for microhematuria and graft dysfunction through urinalysis, initially at baseline, then quarterly for the first year, and subsequently annually. If recurrence is suspected, an allograft biopsy is recommended for confirmation and to rule out other potential causes [16,95,102].

2.2.6. Lupus Nephritis (LN)

Prevalence and Time to Recurrence: Recurrent lupus nephritis (RLN) after kidney transplantation varies widely, from 2.44% in registry analyses [108] to 30–54% in single-center reports [109]. This is due to differing biopsy practices (for-cause vs. protocol), follow-up duration, population, and immunosuppressive regimens [108,110,111]. RLN can occur anytime, from one week to 16 years post-transplant, though most events occur within 10 years. Patient demographics, ANA, dsDNA, and complement activity are poor relapse markers; new-onset proteinuria and hematuria are the clinical indicators of biopsy.

Graft Outcome: Severe RLN, though uncommon, raises graft failure risk significantly; one study showed 93% failure with RLN versus 19% in controls, and a fourfold greater risk than without recurrence [108]. However, RLN accounts for only 7% of overall graft failure, compared to 43% for rejection. Patient survival rates are similar for RLN and rejection patients, and not notably lower than controls without recurrence [108].

Risk Factors:

- Recipient Factors: Non-Hispanic Black race, female gender, age <33, dialysis pre-transplant [108], and the presence of antiphospholipid antibodies [109,112]. High SLEDAI or serologic activity at transplant may also increase risk, though the American College of Rheumatology (ACR) states that serologic activity alone should not preclude transplantation [111].
- Donor Factors: Recipients of RLN commonly received a deceased-donor kidney allograft. High levels of HLA-A and HLA-B locus mismatch in deceased-donor transplants, and a high frequency of zero-haplotype match with living donors, are also associated with increased risk [108]. Some studies suggest a higher recurrence rate with living donor kidneys, though this finding is not consistent across all cohorts [109].
- Immunosuppression: Mycophenolate reduces RLN incidence [108]. Though maintenance azathioprine hinted at a non-significant trend towards higher risk, the type of induction or maintenance immunosuppression was not a strong independent predictor in multivariate analyses [108]. Lack of induction therapy correlates with increased recurrence and poorer outcomes in some studies [113,114].

Immunological and Pathological Mechanisms:

Recurrent lupus nephritis (RLN) after kidney transplant is caused by the reactivation of systemic autoimmunity, leading to immune complex deposition in the allograft, driven by autoantibodies (such as anti-dsDNA), hypocomplementemia, and immune complex-mediated glomerular injury. Post-transplant immunosuppression usually keeps recurrence low and mild. However, recurrence can happen in patients with active serology at transplant (elevated dsDNA and low complement) or inadequate immunosuppression [114,115]. KDIGO [110] and ACR Guidelines [111] recommend regular monitoring due to potential subclinical recurrence and the risk of extrarenal SLE flares. Non-immune complex mechanisms, such as thrombotic microangiopathy and atypical pauci-immune proliferative GN and FSGS [116], also contribute. Overall, recurrent LN is influenced by persistent autoimmunity and immunosuppression, with most recurrences subclinical and rarely causing graft loss.

Treatment of Recurrent LN (RLN) Post-Kidney Transplantation

RLN post-transplant is managed by adjusting or escalating baseline immunosuppression. This typically involves a calcineurin inhibitor (CNI), mycophenolate, and pulse glucocorticoids, tailored to the lupus nephritis (LN) class, severity, and prior treatment response. For severe or refractory cases, treatment may escalate to triple therapy: glucocorticoids, mycophenolic acid (MPA), and either belimumab or a CNI, or cyclophosphamide and belimumab. If MPA is ineffective, cyclophosphamide may be considered. Rituximab may be added for refractory cases. Intensified immunosuppression generally continues for 3–5 years after a complete renal response before tapering. It is important to note that most of the treatment data for LN is derived from native kidney disease [110,111,117].

Before intensifying immunosuppression, guidelines from the ACR [111] and KDIGO [110] recommend a repeat kidney biopsy. This is crucial to differentiate active lupus nephritis (LN) from chronic allograft injury or other causes of kidney dysfunction. Additionally, supportive therapies like RAAS inhibitors and hydroxychloroquine should be continued as appropriate, unless there are contraindications.

Screening and monitoring of recurrent lupus nephritis: Monitoring for RLN requires regular clinical and laboratory monitoring, including renal function, urinalysis, UPCR, and serologic markers such as dsDNA and complement (with clinical correlation). ACR [111] and KDIGO [110] emphasize follow-up due to the risk of recurrence, although this risk is low, and flares are often mild. Persistent renal abnormalities warrant biopsy to distinguish lupus nephritis from allograft injury. Protocol biopsies are not routinely recommended, although they can detect subclinical recurrences; most centers prefer indication biopsies.

2.2.7. ANCA-Associated Vasculitis (AAV)

Prevalence and Time to Recurrence: The recurrence of AAV in kidney allografts is estimated at 0.1 per patient per year, with both early and late recurrences. Early recurrence (within weeks) causes primary graft non-function and extrarenal symptoms; high seropositivity was linked to recurrence despite clinical remission. Late recurrence, years post-transplantation, had an insidious course, making diagnosis challenging despite multiple kidney biopsies, and progressed to ESRD [118].

Graft Outcome:

AAV recurrence post-transplant is rare (<10%), typically occurring beyond the first post-transplant year. Risk factors (pre-transplant course, ANCA subtype/titer, donor type) are not well-established predictors of recurrence. Though rare, recurrence threatens graft survival and necessitates prompt management. Graft loss more often stems from death with a functioning graft, commonly due to immunosuppression-related infection and malignancy, and not disease recurrence [10,119–121].

Risk Factors:

- Immunological Factors: Persistent post-transplant ANCA modestly elevates risk but is not a strong relapse predictor without confirmation of active disease and does not warrant immunosuppression escalation. ANCA positivity should not delay transplant or impact relapse rates. Close monitoring is recommended for patients with persistently positive titers [95,122].
- Donor Factors: Donor factors (type, age, sex, HLA matching) do not significantly influence AAV recurrence risk after kidney transplantation [10,122,123].
- Recipient Factors: Recipient age, disease duration, and comorbidities do not significantly influence AAV recurrence risk post-transplant [122].
- Immunosuppression: Modern regimens (calcineurin inhibitors, mycophenolate mofetil, corticosteroids) reduce relapse rates [121]; standard protocols are recommended, and prophylactic immunosuppression with RTX is not recommended.
- Timing of Transplant: Receiving the transplant while ANCA vasculitis is still active carries a high risk of recurrence and mortality, especially PR3 positivity [53]. Persistent ANCA should not delay transplantation. Guidelines recommend delaying kidney transplantation until patients are in complete remission for at least 6 months, or ideally 12 months, despite persistent ANCA antibodies [122].

Immunological and Pathological Mechanisms: AAV recurrence after kidney transplant results from reactivated autoimmunity against neutrophil antigens (PR3, MPO), causing pauci-immune necrotizing and crescentic glomerulonephritis in the allograft, sometimes accompanied by arteritis or granulomatous vasculitis. Persistent ANCA drives recurrence by activating neutrophils/monocytes, leading to endothelial injury and small-vessel vasculitis. Theories for recurrence include incomplete T-helper cell inhibition by transplant immunosuppressants and epitope spreading beyond PR3/MPO [10,120].

Histology

Clinical presentations often include rising serum creatinine, hematuria, and proteinuria and rising ANCA titers. Histopathologically, recurrence is characterized by pauci-immune necrotizing and crescentic glomerulonephritis, and may also present as acute arteritis or, rarely, granulomatous vasculitis, causing ureteral stenosis or obstructive uropathy. Biopsy is essential to confirm active disease, distinguish recurrence from chronic injury or rejection, and guide therapy [10,122].

Treatment of AAV Recurrence Post-Kidney Transplantation

Rapid reinduction of remission is critical. High-dose glucocorticoids are the cornerstone of initial therapy due to the risk of rapid allograft loss if vasculitis is uncontrolled. Rituximab is preferred for relapsing AAV post-transplant due to its efficacy and favorable safety profile compared to cyclophosphamide, especially with prior cyclophosphamide exposure [120,124,125]. KDIGO 2024 guidelines recommend rituximab first-line for relapsing/refractory disease, with cyclophosphamide as an alternative [95,122]. Plasma exchange may be added for severe/refractory, life-threatening cases [122,126].

Managing refractory disease may involve switching rituximab/cyclophosphamide, increasing glucocorticoids, or adding plasma exchange, tailored to patient factors like prior drug exposure, comorbidities, and infection risk. Evidence in transplant patients is limited, relying on native kidney disease data and small case series; further research is needed [122].

Screening and monitoring of AAV recurrence: Post-kidney transplant, AAV recurrence requires close clinical surveillance, including structured assessments, inflammatory markers, and kidney function tests (eGFR, creatinine, proteinuria, hematuria). Recurrence risk is low, but vigilant monitoring is crucial, as relapses can occur later and present as pauci-immune GN or extrarenal relapses. While routine ANCA titer monitoring can be performed, changes are only modestly predictive of relapse and should not be the sole guide. Persistent or rising ANCA, especially in PR3-ANCA patients, may necessitate closer observation, but ANCA positivity at transplant does not reliably predict recurrence. There is no consensus on monitoring frequency, but continuous vigilance for clinical and lab evidence of recurrence is recommended. If suspected, prompt evaluation (including kidney biopsy and consideration of reinduction with rituximab) is advised [95,122].

3. Conclusions

Recurrent GN post-kidney transplant remains a challenge in transplant nephrology. Transplantation improves ESRD patient survival and quality of life but does not cure the underlying systemic disease that initially caused kidney failure. Therefore, the allograft is susceptible to GN recurrence, affecting long-term graft survival.

Post-transplant GN recurrence varies greatly by subtype, from rare in anti-GBM to almost universal in DDD, emphasizing the need for accurate pre-transplant diagnosis and risk stratification. FSGS and MPGN/C3G carry high recurrence and early graft loss risks. IgAN frequently recurs but has better long-term graft outcomes. Lupus nephritis and AAV have lower recurrence rates in allografts; graft loss is often due to immunosuppression complications (infection, malignancy) rather than direct disease recurrence. The risk of recurrence of 3–15% is an underestimate. A total of 45% of allografts fail within 5 years of recurrence [3,6–8], and recurrent GN is the third leading cause of graft loss at 10 years. Recurrent GN diagnosis hinges on clinical suspicion (proteinuria, hematuria, declining graft function) and renal allograft biopsy (light microscopy, immunofluorescence, electron microscopy). While "for-cause" biopsies are common, "protocol" biopsies reveal more subclinical recurrences and a higher true incidence. Monitoring strategies are GN subtype-specific, using serological markers and varied clinical/lab assessments.

Recurrence mechanisms are diverse, often involving persistent circulating factors in FSGS, autoantibodies (PLA2R in MN, anti-dsDNA in RLN, ANCA in AAV), or complement dysregulation in C3G. Genetic predispositions are key in IgAN and C3G. Recurrence risk factors include recipient characteristics (younger age, rapid progression to ESRD, prior recurrence), immunological markers (antibody titers, complement levels, presence of monoclonal gammopathy), and aspects of transplant management (e.g., immunosuppressive regimens, type of donor).

This narrative review has several limitations, including potential selection bias due to non-systematic study inclusion and possible omission of relevant studies. A formal risk-of-bias assessment or meta-analysis was not performed, so findings should be interpreted with caution. The evidence base is heterogeneous across diseases and study designs, with variability in diagnostic criteria and outcome definitions. Most data are derived from retrospective cohorts and transplant registries, which are subject to indication and survivorship biases. Across subtypes, outcome reporting is inconsistent, and response criteria are not standardized in the transplant setting. Randomized controlled trials specifically in kidney transplant recipients are scarce, and the generalizability from native kidney disease studies is uncertain. Future efforts should focus on developing and validating predictive biomarkers for recurrence risk stratification pre- and post-transplant by disease subtype. It is also important to establish standardized diagnostic and response criteria tailored to the transplant context, including biopsy and non-invasive markers. Conducting multicenter prospective cohorts and pragmatic trials to evaluate therapies and monitoring strategies in transplant recipients and creating shared registries with harmonized data elements to enable comparative effectiveness analyses across centers would also be beneficial.

In conclusion, the recurrence of GN post-kidney transplantation is a complex and significant determinant of long-term graft success. The differential impact of recurrence across GN subtypes necessitates highly individualized patient management, from pre-transplant counseling and risk assessment to tailored immunosuppression and vigilant post-transplant monitoring. Continued research into the precise immunopathogenesis of each GN type, the identification of reliable predictive biomarkers, and the development of targeted therapeutic interventions are paramount to improving outcomes for kidney transplant recipients facing this persistent challenge.

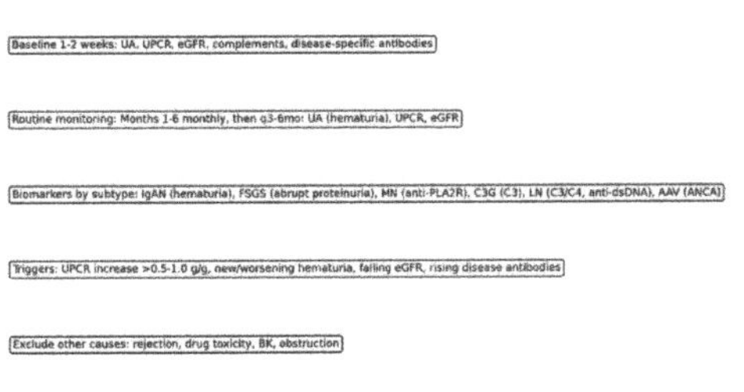

Figure 1. Monitoring algorithm for post-transplant surveillance and biopsy thresholds by subtype.

Table 1. Incidence and time to recurrence by GN subtypes.

Subtype	Reported Recurrence Rate	Time to Recurrence	Impact on Graft Survival
Overall recurrent GN	3–15% (likely an underestimate).	Increases with time; the 2nd most common biopsy finding at 10 years.	45% of grafts fail within 5 years of recurrence [3,6–8]; 3rd leading cause of graft loss at 10 years.
IgA nephropathy (IgAN)	10–30% (indication biopsy); 25–53% (protocol biopsy) [9–12]; up to 51% at 5 years.	Median ~59 months (range 16–90 months); clinical recurrence often after 5 years.	Graft loss in up to 40%; ~42% 5–year graft failure; accounts for 60% of graft failures in this group.
FSGS	Recurrence 40–60%; up to 80% in high-risk cohorts [37].	Recurrence often occurs within days to months (median 1.5 months) post-transplant, mostly within the first two years [36,37].	Recurrent FSGS significantly reduces 5-year graft survival to 52%, compared to 83% in non-recurrent cases, with most graft losses occurring within two years of recurrence. De novo FSGS offers better long-term graft survival (60%) than recurrent FSGS (33.3%), with slower progression [38].
Membranous nephropathy	10–45%, 31% incidence at 10 years.	Median 6.3 years, longer than other GN. Early recurrence (6–12 months) suggests pre-existing antibodies; late onset (~5 years) implies new antibody production.	Better in recurrent membranous nephropathy compared to de novo (11.7/100 person-years vs. 3.7/100 person-years [68]).
MPGN/C3 glomerulopathy (C3G, DDD)	C3G and monoclonal IC-MPGN have 20–50% higher recurrence rates, with C3G exceeding 60–70%. DDD almost always recurs (near 100%).	C3G often recurs early post-transplant [37,82,83], sometimes within 9 days (median 1.1–28 months) [84].	Recurrent MPGN and C3G lead to poor graft outcomes, with C3G recurrence causing graft failure in 11–77% (mostly >50%) [82–86]. Graft loss is more frequent and rapid in DDD than in C3 glomerulonephritis [84].
Anti-GBM disease	Rare 1.9–4% [104].	Early recurrence is related to circulating antibodies at transplant.	Post-transplant GN recurrence is rare, but links to graft loss. Overall, patient and graft survival are excellent, and atypical anti-GBM outcomes are favorable.
Lupus nephritis (LN)	2.44% in registry analyses [108] (high as 30–54% in single-center cohorts based on biopsy patterns [109]).	1 week to several years, most within 10 years.	Rarely causes graft loss (7%); severe LN is uncommon but has higher graft loss. One study revealed 93% failure with RLN versus 19% in controls, and a fourfold greater risk than without recurrence [108].
ANCA-associated vasculitis	Rare, 0.1 per patient per year, with both early and late recurrences.	Early recurrence (weeks) leads to primary graft non-function and extrarenal symptoms. Late recurrence (years) is insidious, hard to diagnose, and progresses to ESRD despite biopsies [118].	Graft loss often results from death with a functioning graft, frequently due to immunosuppression-related infection and malignancy, not disease recurrence [10,119–121].

Table 2. Risk factors for recurrent GN after kidney transplantation.

Subtype	Risk Factors
IgA nephropathy	Risk factors for post-transplant IgAN recurrence include younger age at diagnosis/transplant [9,15], rapid ESRD progression, prior transplant, pre-transplant hemodialysis [15], steroid withdrawal/sparing, mTOR inhibitor use [15,17], elevated Gd-IgA1 and anti-Gd-IgA1 [18], low HLA-DR mismatch [15], living donor status, crescentic disease, rapid pre-transplant eGFR decline [20], and presence of pre/post-transplant DSAs [9].
FSGS	Risk factors for recurrent FSGS include younger age, rapid progression to ESRD [39,40], white race, pre-transplant antinephrin antibodies [41,42], prior recurrent FSGS (80% risk), and nephrotic syndrome at native disease onset [39,40].
Membranous nephropathy	Risk factors include elevated anti-PLA2R pre-transplant [7,37,71–73], female sex, younger age [5], recipient HLA-A3, living-related transplants [68], high pre-transplant proteinuria [72], faster ESRD progression [71], and donor HLA-D and PLA2R1 risk alleles [74,75].
MPGN/C3G	Pre-transplant low complement, monoclonal gammopathy [1,53,82], C3 nephritic factor, and genetic abnormalities (CFH, CFI, MCP) [53,84,89,90] are risk factors. Other factors include young age, crescents in original biopsy, low BMI [10,85], shorter dialysis duration before kidney transplantation [87], and prior graft loss from MPGN [10].
Anti-GBM disease	Pre-transplant circulating antibodies [104] and post-transplant cessation or reduction in immunosuppression [104] may lead to recurrence. Factors like pre-transplant disease course, time to transplant, or donor type do not predict recurrence [10,85].
Lupus nephritis	Risk factors include African American or Hispanic ethnicity, younger age, antiphospholipid antibodies [109,112], pre-transplant dialysis [108], HLA-A and HLA-B locus mismatch (deceased-donor), high frequency of zero-haplotype match (living donors) [108], and lack of induction therapy [113,114]. MMF induction reduces recurrence [108].
ANCA-associated vasculitis	Increased post-transplant ANCA titers do not strongly predict relapses or warrant immunosuppression escalation. CNI, MMF, and steroids reduce relapse risk [121]. Donor factors [10,122,123] (type, age, sex, HLA matching), recipient age, disease duration, and comorbidities do not significantly influence AAV recurrence risk [122]. Active ANCA vasculitis at transplant, especially PR3 positivity, carries a high risk of recurrence and mortality. Persistent ANCA should not delay transplantation; guidelines recommend delaying until complete remission for 6–12 months despite persistent ANCA antibodies [122].

Table 3. Management and prognosis of recurrent GN after kidney transplantation.

Subtype	Management Strategies	Prognosis
IgA nephropathy	Supportive therapy includes RAAS blockade [10] and maintaining corticosteroids, avoiding early steroid withdrawal. For active/severe recurrence, IV MP (500 mg daily or 3 days at months 1, 3, 5) combined with oral prednisone (0.5 mg/kg every other day for six months) may be considered [23]. Experimental treatments for severe/treatment-resistant cases (especially with endocapillary proliferation or crescentic lesions) include cyclophosphamide [24–26], rituximab [27,28], and eculizumab [29]. Tonsillectomy is reported to be beneficial in Japan [30]. Novel IgAN therapies (BAFF–APRIL inhibitors) are under investigation [32,33].	Frequent recurrence but relatively favorable compared with other GN [5,9,10,13,14]; graft loss in up to 40%.
FSGS	First-line treatment: plasmapheresis ± rituximab [39] (early RTX benefit), high-dose steroids, intensified calcineurin inhibitors (cyclosporine/tacrolimus). For PLEX or RTX unresponsive cases: ACTH gel [61,62], LDL pheresis [63–65], abatacept, and ofatumumab [66,67].	Early/treatment-resistant recurrence of FSGS has a poor prognosis, with up to 50% graft loss. De novo FSGS offers better graft survival (60%) than recurrent FSGS (33.3%) [38].
Membranous Nephropathy	Adhere to existing transplant immunosuppressants and antiproteinuric agents. Rituximab is preferred first-line immunosuppression [71,72,78], while obinutuzumab has been used for rituximab-resistant recurrent MN in case reports and series [79–81].	Favorable outcome with graft survival.
MPGN/C3G	For IC-MPGN, glucocorticoids are the initial immunosuppressants. Mycophenolate mofetil, rituximab [92,93], or cyclophosphamide [94] are alternatives if glucocorticoids are contraindicated, not tolerated, or ineffective; complement inhibition (eculizumab, ravulizumab) in C3G/DDD; Iptacopan [97] and pegcetacoplan in C3G have shown promise [98,99]; supportive therapy with RAAS blockade; treatment of underlying disease.	High recurrence, poor graft survival, especially in DDD.
Anti-GBM disease	High-dose corticosteroids, daily PLEX (until antibody titers negative), and oral cyclophosphamide are primary treatments. Rituximab may benefit refractory cases.	Recurrence is rare but associated with graft loss.
Lupus nephritis	Standard immunosuppression (steroids, MMF, calcineurin inhibitors) should be maintained and escalated as needed. Post-transplant, add hydroxychloroquine. For refractory disease, consider cyclophosphamide, belimumab, or rituximab.	Generally indolent; rarely causes graft failure; outcomes favorable with adequate immunosuppression.
ANCA-associated vasculitis	High-dose corticosteroids; rituximab preferred over cyclophosphamide for relapsing disease. PLEX for life-threatening cases.	Good prognosis with early recognition and treatment.

Table 4. Screening and monitoring for the risk of recurrence.

Disease	Key Monitoring Parameters and Tests	Recommended Frequency	Biopsy Guidance and Key Notes
IgA Nephropathy (IgAN)	Urine for microhematuria, proteinuria, creatinine, and eGFR	Monthly for the 1st month, then quarterly for the 1st year, then annually.	Kidney biopsy is indicated for new/worsening disease or graft dysfunction [10,16]. Investigational biomarkers (e.g., Gd-IgA1) are not standard.
Recurrent FSGS (rFSGS)	Proteinuria (spot urine UPCR/UACR), creatinine, eGFR	High-Risk Patients: Daily for 1 week, weekly for 4 weeks, quarterly for 1 year, then annually.	Recurrence is confirmed by kidney biopsy [10,16]. Pre-transplant genetic testing is vital to exclude genetic forms. Investigational biomarkers include suPAR, CLC-1, AT1R-Ab, anti-CD40, IL-13, and antinephrin antibodies.
Recurrent Membranous Nephropathy (MN)	Proteinuria (spot urine UPCR/UACR), creatinine, eGFR, anti-PLA2R antibodies (if PLA2R-positive MN)	Proteinuria: Monthly for 6–12 months. Anti-PLA2R: Monthly to quarterly, per pre-transplant levels.	Kidney biopsy indicated for proteinuria >1 g/day or rising anti-PLA2R (0.3–1.0 g/day) [71,78]. For non-PLA2R MN, biopsy if proteinuria >1 g/day [78].
MPGN/C3G	Proteinuria (spot urine UPCR/UACR), eGFR/creatinine, hematuria, Complement levels (C3, C4) with monoclonal protein screening	No single standard protocol exists; monitoring is regular but individualized based on the patient's case.	First 1–2 years post-transplant, surveillance biopsies are highly recommended due to potential subclinical recurrence [101,102]. Prompt biopsies are vital for unexplained graft dysfunction, new/worsening proteinuria, or hematuria. Complement biomarker profiling and genetic testing are considered in specific cases for prognosis and therapy. Despite guidelines, no standardized protocol exists; monitoring is individualized based on risk factors, disease subtype, and evolving evidence [37,88,103].
Anti-GBM Disease	Urinalysis (for microhematuria) and graft function (eGFR, creatinine)	Quarterly for the 1st year, then annually.	Kidney biopsy is recommended to confirm a suspected recurrence [16,95,102].
Lupus Nephritis (RLN)	Kidney function (eGFR/creatinine) Urinalysis/UPCR Inflammatory markers (CRP, ESR) Serologic markers (dsDNA, complement)	Regular, long-term monitoring is required, but a specific schedule is not standardized.	ACR [111] and KDIGO [110] highlight the importance of follow-up for recurrence risk, despite it being low and flares usually mild. Persistent renal abnormalities require biopsy to differentiate lupus nephritis from allograft injury. Protocol biopsies are not standard; indication biopsies are preferred.
ANCA-Associated Vasculitis (AAV)	Kidney function (eGFR/creatinine) and urinalysis (for hematuria and proteinuria), inflammatory markers (CRP and ESR), ANCA titers	No consensus on frequency; requires continuous clinical vigilance.	Kidney Biopsy: Advised for prompt evaluation if recurrence is suspected [95,122]. Notes: ANCA levels alone are not reliable predictors of relapse.

Author Contributions: Conceptualization, A.K., A.S. and D.G.; Methodology, A.K., A.S. and D.G.; Writing, A.K., A.S. and D.G.; Supervision, D.G. All authors have read and agreed to the published version of the manuscript.

Funding: This review paper received no external funding.

Data Availability Statement: No new data were created or analyzed in this study as this is a narrative review. All the references have been listed. Data sharing is not applicable to this article.

Conflicts of Interest: A. Koirala serves on the advisory board for Calliditas Pharmaceuticals, focusing on targeted release budesonide. While this relationship is disclosed for transparency, A. Koirala asserts that it did not influence the content, analysis, or conclusions of this review paper. Duvuru Geetha has received consultancy fees from Calliditas, Vera therapeutics, Travere therapeutics, Amgen, Otsuka and Boeringer Ingelheim. The authors declare no conflict of interest for the review paper.

Abbreviations

AAV	ANCA-associated vasculitis
DDD	dense deposit disease
ESRD	end-stage kidney disease
FSGS	focal segmental glomerulosclerosis
GBM	glomerular basement membrane
GN	glomerulonephritis/glomerular diseases
KDIGO	Kidney Disease: Improving Global Outcomes
LN	lupus nephritis
MMF	mycophenolate mofetil
MN	membranous nephropathy
MPGN	membranoproliferative glomerulonephritis
RAAS	renin–angiotensin–aldosterone system

References

1. Lim, W.H.; Shingde, M.; Wong, G. Recurrent and de novo Glomerulonephritis After Kidney Transplantation. *Front. Immunol.* **2019**, *10*, 1944. [CrossRef]
2. Salvadori, M.; Rosso, G. Recurrence of primary glomerular diseases after kidney transplantation: Incidence, predictors, characteristics and treatment. *Transplantology* **2025**, *6*, 14. [CrossRef]
3. Mayrdorfer, M.; Liefeldt, L.; Wu, K.; Rudolph, B.; Zhang, Q.; Friedersdorff, F.; Lachmann, N.; Schmidt, D.; Osmanodja, B.; Naik, M.G.; et al. Exploring the complexity of death-censored kidney allograft failure. *J. Am. Soc. Nephrol.* **2021**, *32*, 1513–1526. [CrossRef] [PubMed]
4. Saran, R.; Robinson, B.; Abbott, K.C.; Bragg-Gresham, J.; Chen, X.; Gipson, D.; Gu, H.; Hirth, R.A.; Hutton, D.; Jin, Y.; et al. US renal data system 2019 annual data report: Epidemiology of kidney disease in the United States. *Am. J. Kidney Dis.* **2020**, *75* (Suppl. 1), A6–A7. [CrossRef] [PubMed]
5. Allen, P.J.; Chadban, S.J.; Craig, J.C.; Lim, W.H.; Allen, R.D.M.; Clayton, P.A.; Teixeira-Pinto, A.; Wong, G. Recurrent glomerulonephritis after kidney transplantation: Risk factors and allograft outcomes. *Kidney Int.* **2017**, *92*, 461–469. [CrossRef] [PubMed]
6. Aguiar, R.; Bourmpaki, E.; Bunce, C.; Coker, B.; Delaney, F.; de Jongh, L.; Oliveira, G.; Weir, A.; Higgins, F.; Spiridou, A.; et al. Incidence, Risk Factors, and Effect on Allograft Survival of Glomerulonephritis Post-transplantation in a United Kingdom Population: Cohort Study. *Front. Nephrol.* **2022**, *2*, 923813. [CrossRef]
7. Jiang, S.H.; Kennard, A.L.; Walters, G.D. Recurrent glomerulonephritis following renal transplantation and impact on graft survival. *BMC Nephrol.* **2018**, *19*, 344. [CrossRef]
8. Alawieh, R.; Boonpheng, B.; Blosser, C.D. Recurrence of glomerulonephritis after kidney transplant. *Nephrol. Dial. Transplant.* **2022**, *37*, 2090–2092. [CrossRef]
9. Uffing, A.; Pérez-Saéz, M.J.; Jouve, T.; Bugnazet, M.; Malvezzi, P.; Muhsin, S.A.; Lafargue, M.-C.; Reindl-Schwaighofer, R.; Morlock, A.; Oberbauer, R.; et al. Recurrence of IgA nephropathy after kidney transplantation in adults. *Clin. J. Am. Soc. Nephrol.* **2021**, *16*, 1247–1255. [CrossRef]
10. Kidney Disease: Improving Global Outcomes (KDIGO); Transplant Work Group. KDIGO clinical practice guideline for the care of kidney transplant recipients. *Am. J. Transplant.* **2009**, *9* (Suppl. 3), S1–S155. [CrossRef]

11. Kawabe, M.; Yamamoto, I. Current status and perspectives on recurrent IgA nephropathy after kidney transplantation. *Nephron* **2023**, *147* (Suppl. 1), 9–13. [CrossRef] [PubMed]
12. Jäger, C.; Stampf, S.; Molyneux, K.; Barratt, J.; Golshayan, D.; Hadaya, K.; Huynh-Do, U.; Binet, F.-I.; Mueller, T.F.; Koller, M.; et al. Recurrence of IgA nephropathy after kidney transplantation: Experience from the Swiss transplant cohort study. *BMC Nephrol.* **2022**, *23*, 178. [CrossRef] [PubMed]
13. Engen, R.M.; Bartosh, S.M.; Smith, J.M.; Perkins, J.D.; Harshman, L.A. Risk for graft loss in pediatric and young adult kidney transplant recipients due to recurrent IgA nephropathy. *Am. J. Transplant.* **2024**, *24*, 37–45. [CrossRef] [PubMed]
14. Bednarova, K.; Mjøen, G.; Hruba, P.; Modos, I.; Voska, L.; Kollar, M.; Viklicky, O. A novel prognostic nomogram predicts premature failure of kidney allografts with IgA nephropathy recurrence. *Nephrol. Dial. Transplant.* **2023**, *38*, 2627–2636. [CrossRef]
15. Li, Y.; Tang, Y.; Lin, T.; Song, T. Risk factors and outcomes of IgA nephropathy recurrence after kidney transplantation: A systematic review and meta-analysis. *Front. Immunol.* **2023**, *14*, 1277017. [CrossRef]
16. Bia, M.; Adey, D.B.; Bloom, R.D.; Chan, L.; Kulkarni, S.; Tomlanovich, S. KDOQI US commentary on the 2009 KDIGO clinical practice guideline for the care of kidney transplant recipients. *Am. J. Kidney Dis.* **2010**, *56*, 189–218. [CrossRef]
17. Lionaki, S.; Makropoulos, I.; Panagiotellis, K.; Vlachopanos, G.; Gavalas, I.; Marinaki, S.; Liapis, G.; Michelakis, I.; Bokos, I.; Boletis, I.; et al. Kidney transplantation outcomes in patients with IgA nephropathy and other glomerular and non-glomerular primary diseases in the new era of immunosuppression. *PLoS ONE* **2021**, *16*, e0253337. [CrossRef]
18. Berthelot, L.; Robert, T.; Vuiblet, V.; Tabary, T.; Braconnier, A.; Dramé, M.; Toupance, O.; Rieu, P.; Monteiro, R.C.; Touré, F. Recurrent IgA nephropathy is predicted by altered glycosylated IgA, autoantibodies and soluble CD89 complexes. *Kidney Int.* **2015**, *88*, 815–822. [CrossRef]
19. Garnier, A.-S.; Duveau, A.; Demiselle, J.; Croué, A.; Subra, J.-F.; Sayegh, J.; Augusto, J.-F.; Moura, I.C. Early post-transplant serum IgA level is associated with IgA nephropathy recurrence after kidney transplantation. *PLoS ONE* **2018**, *13*, e0196101. [CrossRef]
20. Maixnerova, D.; Hruba, P.; Neprasova, M.; Bednarova, K.; Slatinska, J.; Suchanek, M.; Kollar, M.; Novak, J.; Tesar, V.; Viklicky, O. Outcome of 313 Czech patients with IgA nephropathy after renal transplantation. *Front. Immunol.* **2021**, *12*, 726215. [CrossRef]
21. Moroni, G.; Belingheri, M.; Frontini, G.; Tamborini, F.; Messa, P. Immunoglobulin A Nephropathy. Recurrence After Renal Transplantation. *Front. Immunol.* **2019**, *10*, 1332. [CrossRef] [PubMed]
22. Ong, S.C.; Julian, B.A. Post-transplant IgA Nephropathy. *Semin. Nephrol.* **2024**, *44*, 151570. [CrossRef] [PubMed]
23. Messina, M.; di Vico, M.C.; Ariaudo, C.; Mazzucco, G.; Fop, F.; Segoloni, G.P.; Biancone, L. Treatment protocol with pulse and oral steroids for IgA Nephropathy after kidney transplantation. *J. Nephrol.* **2016**, *29*, 575–583. [CrossRef] [PubMed]
24. Malhotra, P.S.; Jorna, T.; Bhandari, S. Treatment of immunoglobulin A nephropathy recurrence post–renal transplant. *Transplant. Proc.* **2018**, *50*, 165–167. [CrossRef]
25. Tumlin, J.A.; Lohavichan, V.; Hennigar, R. Crescentic, proliferative IgA nephropathy: Clinical and histological response to methylprednisolone and intravenous cyclophosphamide. *Nephrol. Dial. Transplant.* **2003**, *18*, 1321–1329. [CrossRef]
26. Roccatello, D.; Ferro, M.; Cesano, G.; Rossi, D.; Berutti, S.; Salomone, M.; Piccoli, G.; Sena, L.M. Steroid and cyclophosphamide in IgA nephropathy. *Nephrol. Dial. Transplant.* **2000**, *15*, 833–835. [CrossRef]
27. Chancharoenthana, W.; Leelahavanichkul, A.; Ariyanon, W.; Vadcharavivad, S.; Phumratanaprapin, W. Comparative long-term renal allograft outcomes of recurrent immunoglobulin A with severe activity in kidney transplant recipients with and without rituximab: An observational cohort study. *J. Clin. Med.* **2021**, *10*, 3939. [CrossRef]
28. Chancharoenthana, W.; Townamchai, N.; Leelahavanichkul, A.; Wattanatorn, S.; Kanjanabuch, T.; Avihingsanon, Y.; Praditpornsilpa, K.; Eiam-Ong, S. Rituximab for recurrent IgA nephropathy in kidney transplantation: A report of three cases and proposed mechanisms. *Nephrology* **2017**, *22*, 65–71. [CrossRef]
29. Duval, A.; Olagne, J.; Obrecht, A.; Vargas, G.G.; Perrin, P.; Moulin, B.; Frémeaux-Bacchi, V.; Caillard, S. Eculizumab as a therapeutic approach for severe crescentic recurrence of immunoglobulin A nephropathy after kidney transplantation. *Am. J. Transplant.* **2023**, *23*, 1626–1630. [CrossRef]
30. Kawabe, M.; Yamamoto, I.; Yamakawa, T.; Katsumata, H.; Isaka, N.; Katsuma, A.; Koike, K.; Ueda, H. Association between galactose-deficient IgA1 derived from the tonsils and recurrence of IgA nephropathy in patients who underwent kidney transplantation. *Front. Immunol.* **2020**, *11*, 2068. [CrossRef]
31. Noguchi, H.; Tsuchimoto, A.; Ueki, K.; Kaku, K.; Okabe, Y.; Nakamura, M. Reduced recurrence of primary IgA nephropathy in kidney transplant recipients receiving everolimus with corticosteroid: A retrospective, single-center study of 135 transplant patients. *Transplant. Proc.* **2020**, *52*, 3118–3124. [CrossRef]
32. Suzuki, Y. B cell targeting in IgA nephropathy. *Nephrology* **2024**, *29* (Suppl. S2), 39–43. [CrossRef] [PubMed]
33. El Karoui, K.; Fervenza, F.C.; De Vriese, A.S. Treatment of IgA Nephropathy: A Rapidly Evolving Field. *J. Am. Soc. Nephrol.* **2024**, *35*, 103–116. [CrossRef] [PubMed]
34. Shabaka, A.; Tato Ribera, A.; Fernández-Juárez, G. Focal segmental glomerulosclerosis: State-of-the-art and clinical perspective. *Nephron* **2020**, *144*, 413–427. [CrossRef] [PubMed]

35. Battelino, N.; Arnol, M.; Kandus, A.; Ponikvar, R.; Novljan, G. Post-transplant recurrence of focal segmental glomerulosclerosis in a child with heterozygous mutations in NPHS1 and NPHS2. *Ther. Apher. Dial.* **2016**, *20*, 312–317. [CrossRef]
36. Kienzl-Wagner, K.; Waldegger, S.; Schneeberger, S. Disease recurrence-the sword of Damocles in kidney transplantation for primary focal segmental glomerulosclerosis. *Front. Immunol.* **2019**, *10*, 1669. [CrossRef]
37. Puttarajappa, C.M.; Schinstock, C.A.; Wu, C.M.; Leca, N.; Kumar, V.; Vasudev, B.S.; Hariharan, S. KDOQI US commentary on the 2020 KDIGO clinical practice guideline on the evaluation and management of candidates for kidney transplantation. *Am. J. Kidney Dis.* **2021**, *77*, 833–856. [CrossRef]
38. Kim, D.K.; Huh, H.; Kim, Y.; Kim, T.; Kim, Y.H.; Choi, B.H.; Lee, H.J.; Kang, M.S.; Kim, S.R.; Lee, D.W.; et al. Recurrent and DE Novo focal segmental glomerulosclerosis after kidney transplantation: Comparison of clinical features and transplant outcomes. *Transplant. Proc.* **2024**, *56*, 1752–1756. [CrossRef]
39. Uffing, A.; Pérez-Sáez, M.J.; Mazzali, M.; Manfro, R.C.; Bauer, A.C.; de Sottomaior Drumond, F.; O'sHaughnessy, M.M.; Cheng, X.S.; Chin, K.-K.; Ventura, C.G.; et al. Recurrence of FSGS after kidney transplantation in adults. *Clin. J. Am. Soc. Nephrol.* **2020**, *15*, 247–256. [CrossRef]
40. Bai, J.; Zhang, T.; Wang, Y.; Cao, J.; Duan, Z.; Ji, L.; Zhou, Y.; Hao, C.; Guo, Q. Incidence and risk factors for recurrent focal segmental glomerulosclerosis after kidney transplantation: A meta-analysis. *Ren. Fail.* **2023**, *45*, 2201341. [CrossRef]
41. Batal, I.; Watts, A.J.B.; Gibier, J.-B.; Hamroun, A.; Top, I.; Provot, F.; Keller, K.; Ye, X.; Fernandez, H.E.; Leal, R.; et al. Pre-transplant anti-nephrin antibodies are specific predictors of recurrent diffuse podocytopathy in the kidney allograft. *Kidney Int.* **2024**, *106*, 749–752. [CrossRef]
42. Shirai, Y.; Miura, K.; Ishizuka, K.; Ando, T.; Kanda, S.; Hashimoto, J.; Hamasaki, Y.; Hotta, K.; Ito, N.; Honda, K.; et al. A multi-institutional study found a possible role of anti-nephrin antibodies in post-transplant focal segmental glomerulosclerosis recurrence. *Kidney Int.* **2024**, *105*, 608–617. [CrossRef]
43. Yao, T.; Udwan, K.; John, R.; Rana, A.; Haghighi, A.; Xu, L.; Hack, S.; Reich, H.N.; Hladunewich, M.A.; Cattran, D.C.; et al. Integration of genetic testing and pathology for the diagnosis of adults with FSGS. *Clin. J. Am. Soc. Nephrol.* **2019**, *14*, 213–223. [CrossRef]
44. De Vriese, A.S.; Sethi, S.; Nath, K.A.; Glassock, R.J.; Fervenza, F.C. Differentiating primary, genetic, and secondary FSGS in adults: A clinicopathologic approach. *J. Am. Soc. Nephrol.* **2018**, *29*, 759–774. [CrossRef]
45. Canaud, G.; Dion, D.; Zuber, J.; Gubler, M.-C.; Sberro, R.; Thervet, E.; Snanoudj, R.; Charbit, M.; Salomon, R.; Martinez, F.; et al. Recurrence of nephrotic syndrome after transplantation in a mixed population of children and adults: Course of glomerular lesions and value of the Columbia classification of histological variants of focal and segmental glomerulosclerosis (FSGS). *Nephrol. Dial. Transplant.* **2010**, *25*, 1321–1328. [CrossRef] [PubMed]
46. Reiser, J.; Nast, C.C.; Alachkar, N. Permeability factors in focal and segmental glomerulosclerosis. *Adv. Chronic Kidney Dis.* **2014**, *21*, 417–421. [CrossRef] [PubMed]
47. Andresdottir, M.B.; Ajubi, N.; Croockewit, S.; Assmann, K.J.; Hibrands, L.B.; Wetzels, J.F. Recurrent focal glomerulosclerosis: Natural course and treatment with plasma exchange. *Nephrol. Dial. Transplant.* **1999**, *14*, 2650–2656. [CrossRef] [PubMed]
48. Savin, V.J.; Sharma, R.; Sharma, M.; McCarthy, E.T.; Swan, S.K.; Ellis, E.; Lovell, H.; Warady, B.; Gunwar, S.; Chonko, A.M.; et al. Circulating factor associated with increased glomerular permeability to albumin in recurrent focal segmental glomerulosclerosis. *N. Engl. J. Med.* **1996**, *334*, 878–883. [CrossRef]
49. Sharma, M.; Sharma, R.; Reddy, S.R.; McCarthy, E.T.; Savin, V.J. Proteinuria after injection of human focal segmental glomerulosclerosis factor. *Transplantation* **2002**, *73*, 366–372. [CrossRef]
50. Wen, Y.; Shah, S.; Campbell, K.N. Molecular mechanisms of proteinuria in focal segmental glomerulosclerosis. *Front. Med.* **2018**, *5*, 98. [CrossRef]
51. Hengel, F.E.; Dehde, S.; Lassé, M.; Zahner, G.; Seifert, L.; Schnarre, A.; Kretz, O.; Demir, F.; Pinnschmidt, H.O.; Grahammer, F.; et al. Autoantibodies Targeting Nephrin in Podocytopathies. *N. Engl. J. Med.* **2024**, *391*, 422–433. [CrossRef]
52. Shu, Y.; Huang, J.; Jiang, L.; Zhang, Y.-M.; Wang, F.; Wang, X.; Meng, L.-Q.; Cheng, X.-Y.; Liu, G.; Wang, S.-X.; et al. Anti-nephrin antibodies in adult Chinese patients with minimal change disease and primary focal segmental glomerulosclerosis. *Kidney Int.* **2025**, *108*, 433–444. [CrossRef]
53. Chadban, S.J.; Ahn, C.; Axelrod, D.A.; Foster, B.J.; Kasiske, B.L.; Kher, V.; Kumar, D.M.; Oberbauer, R.; Pascual, J.; Pilmore, H.L.; et al. Summary of the kidney disease: Improving Global Outcomes (KDIGO) Clinical Practice Guideline on the evaluation and Management of candidates for Kidney Transplantation. *Transplantation* **2020**, *104*, 708–714. [CrossRef] [PubMed]
54. Campise, M.; Favi, E.; Messa, P. Clinical outcomes of prophylactic and therapeutic plasmapheresis in adult deceased-donor kidney transplant recipients with primary focal segmental glomerulosclerosis. *Exp. Clin. Transplant.* **2019**, *17*, 461–469. [CrossRef] [PubMed]
55. Kwon, H.E.; Kim, Y.H.; Lee, S.A.; Lee, J.J.; Ko, Y.; Shin, S.; Jung, J.H.; Sung, F.S.; Baek, C.H.; Kim, H.; et al. Post-operative recurrence of focal segmental glomerulosclerosis according to pre-transplant treatment after kidney transplantation. *BMC Nephrol.* **2023**, *24*, 53. [CrossRef] [PubMed]

56. Boonpheng, B.; Hansrivijit, P.; Thongprayoon, C.; Mao, S.A.; Vaitla, P.K.; Bathini, T.; Choudhury, A.; Kaewput, W.; A Mao, M.; Cheungpasitporn, W. Rituximab or plasmapheresis for prevention of recurrent focal segmental glomerulosclerosis after kidney transplantation: A systematic review and meta-analysis. *World J. Transplant.* **2021**, *11*, 303–319. [CrossRef]
57. Fornoni, A.; Sageshima, J.; Wei, C.; Merscher-Gomez, S.; Aguillon-Prada, R.; Jauregui, A.N.; Li, J.; Mattiazzi, A.; Ciancio, G.; Chen, L.; et al. Rituximab targets podocytes in recurrent focal segmental glomerulosclerosis. *Sci. Transl. Med.* **2011**, *3*, 85ra46. [CrossRef]
58. Kronbichler, A.; Gauckler, P.; Lee, K.H.; Shin, J.I.; Malvezzi, P.; Mayer, G. Immunoadsorption in nephrotic syndrome: Where are we now and where are we going from here? *Atheroscler. Suppl.* **2019**, *40*, 55–60. [CrossRef]
59. Allard, L.; Kwon, T.; Krid, S.; Bacchetta, J.; Garnier, A.; Novo, R.; Deschenes, G.; Salomon, R.; Roussey, G.; Allain-Launay, E. Treatment by immunoadsorption for recurrent focal segmental glomerulosclerosis after paediatric kidney transplantation: A multicentre French cohort. *Nephrol. Dial. Transplant.* **2018**, *33*, 954–963. [CrossRef]
60. Lanaret, C.; Anglicheau, D.; Audard, V.; Büchler, M.; Caillard, S.; Couzi, L.; Malvezzi, P.; Mesnard, L.; Bertrand, D.; Martinez, F.; et al. Rituximab for recurrence of primary focal segmental glomerulosclerosis after kidney transplantation: Results of a nationwide study. *Am. J. Transplant.* **2021**, *21*, 3021–3033. [CrossRef]
61. Alhamad, T.; Manllo Dieck, J.; Younus, U.; Matar, D.; Alasfar, S.; Vujjini, V.; Wall, D.; Kanawati, B.; Reiser, J.; Brennan, D.C.; et al. ACTH gel in resistant focal segmental glomerulosclerosis after kidney transplantation. *Transplantation* **2019**, *103*, 202–209. [CrossRef]
62. Chen, L.; Wu, J.; Ying, D.; Jiang, M.; Xu, Y.; Mo, Y.; Rong, L.; Jiang, X. Application of adrenocorticotropic hormone in recurrent focal segmental glomerulosclerosis post-transplantation: A case report and literature review. *Pediatr. Transplant.* **2022**, *26*, e14184. [CrossRef]
63. Shah, L.; Hooper, D.K.; Okamura, D.; Wallace, D.; Moodalbail, D.; Gluck, C.; Koziell, A.; Zaritsky, J.J. LDL-apheresis-induced remission of focal segmental glomerulosclerosis recurrence in pediatric renal transplant recipients. *Pediatr. Nephrol.* **2019**, *34*, 2343–2350. [CrossRef] [PubMed]
64. Raina, R.; Krishnappa, V. An update on LDL apheresis for nephrotic syndrome. *Pediatr. Nephrol.* **2019**, *34*, 1655–1669. [CrossRef] [PubMed]
65. Gianos, E.; Duell, P.B.; Toth, P.P.; Moriarty, P.M.; Thompson, G.R.; Brinton, E.A.; Hudgins, L.C.; Nametka, M.; Byrne, K.H.; Raghuveer, G.; et al. Lipoprotein apheresis: Utility, outcomes, and implementation in clinical practice: A scientific statement from the American heart association. *Arterioscler. Thromb. Vasc. Biol.* **2024**, *44*, e304–e321. [CrossRef] [PubMed]
66. Reynolds, B.C.; Lamb, A.; Jones, C.A.; Yadav, P.; Tyerman, K.S.; Geddes, C.C. UK experience of ofatumumab in recurrence of focal segmental glomerulosclerosis post-kidney transplant. *Pediatr. Nephrol.* **2022**, *37*, 199–207. [CrossRef]
67. Ural, Z.; Helvacı, Ö.; Özbaş, B.; Güz, G.; Derici, Ü. Unexpected late response to ofatumumab in adult post-transplantation recurrent focal segmental glomerulosclerosis, case report. *Transplant. Proc.* **2022**, *54*, 1632–1635. [CrossRef]
68. Batal, I.; Vasilescu, E.-R.; Dadhania, D.M.; Adel, A.A.; Husain, S.A.; Avasare, R.; Serban, G.; Santoriello, D.; Khairallah, P.; Patel, A.; et al. Association of HLA typing and alloimmunity with posttransplantation membranous nephropathy: A multicenter case series. *Am. J. Kidney Dis.* **2020**, *76*, 374–383. [CrossRef]
69. Ponticelli, C.; Glassock, R.J. De novo membranous nephropathy (MN) in kidney allografts. A peculiar form of alloimmune disease? *Transpl. Int.* **2012**, *25*, 1205–1210. [CrossRef]
70. Panagakis, A.; Bellos, I.; Grigorakos, K.; Panagoutsos, S.; Passadakis, P.; Marinaki, S. Recurrence of idiopathic membranous nephropathy in the kidney allograft: A systematic review. *Biomedicines* **2024**, *12*, 739. [CrossRef]
71. Hullekes, F.; Uffing, A.; Verhoeff, R.; Seeger, H.; von Moos, S.; Mansur, J.; Mastroianni-Kirsztajn, G.; Silva, H.T.; Buxeda, A.; Pérez-Sáez, M.J.; et al. Recurrence of membranous nephropathy after kidney transplantation: A multicenter retrospective cohort study. *Am. J. Transplant.* **2024**, *24*, 1016–1026. [CrossRef]
72. Grupper, A.; Cornell, L.D.; Fervenza, F.C.; Beck, L.H., Jr.; Lorenz, E.; Cosio, F.G. Recurrent membranous nephropathy after kidney transplantation: Treatment and long-term implications. *Transplantation* **2016**, *100*, 2710–2716. [CrossRef]
73. Cremoni, M.; Teisseyre, M.; Thaunat, O.; Fernandez, C.; Payre, C.; Moutou, A.; Zarif, H.; Brglez, V.; Albano, L.; Moal, V.; et al. Anti phospholipase A2 receptor 1 antibodies and membranous nephropathy recurrence after kidney transplantation. *Kidney Int. Rep.* **2024**, *9*, 3427–3438. [CrossRef]
74. Robson, K.J.; Kitching, A.R. Recurrent membranous nephropathy after transplantation: Donor antigen and HLA converge in defining risk. *Kidney Int.* **2021**, *99*, 545–548. [CrossRef] [PubMed]
75. Berchtold, L.; Letouzé, E.; Alexander, M.P.; Canaud, G.; Logt A-Evan de Hamilton, P.; Mousson, C.; Vuiblet, V.; Moyer, A.M.; Guibert, S. HLA-D and PLA2R1 risk alleles associate with recurrent primary membranous nephropathy in kidney transplant recipients. *Kidney Int.* **2021**, *99*, 671–685. [CrossRef] [PubMed]
76. Leon, J.; Pérez-Sáez, M.J.; Batal, I.; Beck, L.H., Jr.; Rennke, H.G.; Canaud, G.; Legendre, C.; Pascual, J.; Riella, L.V. Membranous nephropathy posttransplantation: An update of the pathophysiology and management. *Transplantation* **2019**, *103*, 1990–2002. [CrossRef] [PubMed]
77. Filippone, E.J.; Farber, J.L. Membranous nephropathy in the kidney allograft. *Clin. Transplant.* **2016**, *30*, 1394–1402. [CrossRef]

78. Rovin, B.H.; Adler, S.G.; Barratt, J.; Bridoux, F.; Burdge, K.A.; Chan, T.M.; Cook, H.T.; Fervenza, F.C.; Gibson, K.L.; Glassock, R.J.; et al. KDIGO 2021 Clinical Practice Guideline for the Management of Glomerular Diseases. *Kidney Int.* **2021**, *100*, S1–S276. [CrossRef]
79. Deng, L.; Xu, G. Update on the application of monoclonal antibody therapy in primary membranous nephropathy. *Drugs* **2023**, *83*, 507–530. [CrossRef]
80. Delbet, J.-D.; Hogan, J.; Parmentier, C.; Ulinski, T.; Dossier, C. Successful global anti-B-cell strategy with daratumumab in a patient with post-transplant nephrotic syndrome recurrence unresponsive to immunoadsorption and obinutuzumab. *Pediatr. Transplant.* **2023**, *27*, e14544. [CrossRef]
81. Sethi, S.; Kumar, S.; Lim, K.; Jordan, S.C. Obinutuzumab is effective for the treatment of refractory membranous nephropathy. *Kidney Int. Rep.* **2020**, *5*, 1515–1518. [CrossRef]
82. Alasfar, S.; Carter-Monroe, N.; Rosenberg, A.Z.; Montgomery, R.A.; Alachkar, N. Membranoproliferative glomerulonephritis recurrence after kidney transplantation: Using the new classification. *BMC Nephrol.* **2016**, *17*, 7. [CrossRef]
83. Caravaca-Fontán, F.; Polanco, N.; Villacorta, B.; Buxeda, A.; Coca, A.; Ávila, A.; Martínez-Gallardo, R.; Galeano, C.; Valero, R.; Ramos, N.; et al. Recurrence of immune complex and complement-mediated membranoproliferative glomerulonephritis in kidney transplantation. *Nephrol. Dial. Transplant.* **2023**, *38*, 222–235. [CrossRef] [PubMed]
84. Attieh, R.M.; Bharati, J.; Sharma, P.; Nair, G.; Ayehu, G.; Jhaveri, K.D. Kidney transplant in patients with C3 glomerulopathy. *Clin Kidney J.* **2025**, *18*, sfaf134. [CrossRef] [PubMed]
85. Chukwu, C.A.; Holmberg, C.; Storrar, J.; Middleton, R.; Sinha, S.; Kalra, P.A.; Shawki, H.; Rao, A. Clinical and histopathologic predictors of recurrent glomerulonephritis after kidney transplantation. *Clin. Transplant.* **2023**, *37*, e14970. [CrossRef] [PubMed]
86. Braun, M.C.; Stablein, D.M.; Hamiwka, L.A.; Bell, L.; Bartosh, S.M.; Strife, C.F. Recurrence of membranoproliferative glomerulonephritis type II in renal allografts: The North American Pediatric Renal Transplant Cooperative Study experience. *J. Am. Soc. Nephrol.* **2005**, *16*, 2225–2233. [CrossRef]
87. Green, H.; Rahamimov, R.; Rozen-Zvi, B.; Pertzov, B.; Tobar, A.; Lichtenberg, S.; Gafter, U.; Mor, E. Recurrent membranoproliferative glomerulonephritis type I after kidney transplantation: A 17-year single-center experience. *Transplantation* **2015**, *99*, 1172–1177. [CrossRef]
88. Bartoli, G.; Dello Strologo, A.; Grandaliano, G.; Pesce, F. Updates on C3 glomerulopathy in kidney transplantation: Pathogenesis and treatment options. *Int. J. Mol. Sci.* **2024**, *25*, 6508. [CrossRef]
89. Regunathan-Shenk, R.; Avasare, R.S.; Ahn, W.; Canetta, P.A.; Cohen, D.J.; Appel, G.B.; Bomback, A.S. Kidney transplantation in C3 glomerulopathy: A case series. *Am. J. Kidney Dis.* **2019**, *73*, 316–323. [CrossRef]
90. Garg, N.; Zhang, Y.; Nicholson-Weller, A.; Khankin, E.V.; Borsa, N.G.; Meyer, N.C.; McDermott, S.; Stillman, I.E.; Rennke, H.G.; Smith, R.J.; et al. C3 glomerulonephritis secondary to mutations in factors H and I: Rapid recurrence in deceased donor kidney transplant effectively treated with eculizumab. *Nephrol. Dial. Transplant.* **2018**, *33*, 2260–2265. [CrossRef]
91. Smith, R.J.H.; Appel, G.B.; Blom, A.M.; Cook, H.T.; D'Agati, V.D.; Fakhouri, F.; Fremeaux-Bacchi, V.; Józsi, M.; Kavanagh, D.; Lambris, J.D.; et al. C3 glomerulopathy—Understanding a rare complement-driven renal disease. *Nat. Rev. Nephrol.* **2019**, *15*, 129–143. [CrossRef] [PubMed]
92. Aziz, F.; Singh, T.; Garg, N.; Zhong, W.; Mandelbrot, D. Post-Transplant Idiopathic Immune Complex Membrano-Proliferative Glomerulonephritis: Characteristics And outcomes. *Clin. Nephrol.* **2023**, *99*, 69–77. [CrossRef] [PubMed]
93. Yango, A.F.; Fischbach, B.V.; Ruiz, R.; Mudrovich, S.; Klintmalm, G. Treatment Of Recurrent, Post-Kidney Transplant Membranoproliferative Glomerulonephritis With Plasmapheresis and Rituximab: A Case Report and Literature Review. *Clin. Nephrol.* **2019**, *91*, 52–58. [CrossRef] [PubMed]
94. Lien, Y.H.; Scott, K. Long-term cyclophosphamide treatment for recurrent type I membranoproliferative glomerulonephritis after transplantation. *Am. J. Kidney Dis.* **2000**, *35*, 539–543. [CrossRef]
95. Beck, L.H., Jr.; Ayoub, I.; Caster, D.; Choi, M.J.; Cobb, J.; Geetha, D.; Rheault, M.N.; Wadhwani, S.; Yau, T.; Whittier, W.L. KDOQI US commentary on the 2021 KDIGO Clinical Practice Guideline for the Management of Glomerular Diseases. *Am. J. Kidney Dis.* **2023**, *82*, 121–175. [CrossRef]
96. McCaughan, J.A.; O'Rourke, D.M.; Courtney, A.E. Recurrent dense deposit disease after renal transplantation: An emerging role for complementary therapies. *Am. J. Transplant.* **2012**, *12*, 1046–1051. [CrossRef]
97. Troise, D.; Infante, B.; Mercuri, S.; Rossini, M.; Gesualdo, L.; Stallone, G. Successful management of C3 glomerulopathy recurrence post-kidney transplantation with Iptacopan: A case report. *Int. J. Mol. Sci.* **2025**, *26*, 5053. [CrossRef]
98. Mancuso, M.C.; Cugno, M.; Griffini, S.; Grovetti, E.; Nittoli, T.; Mastrangelo, A.; Tedesco, F.; Montini, G.; Ardissino, G. Efficacy of complement inhibition with pegcetacoplan in children with C3 glomerulopathy. *Pediatr. Nephrol.* **2025**, *40*, 1959–1963. [CrossRef]
99. Guzman, G.L.; Perry, K.W. Pegcetacoplan for the treatment of paediatric C3 glomerulonephritis: A case report. *Nephrology* **2025**, *30*, e70001. [CrossRef]

100. Bomback, A.S.; Daina, E.; Remuzzi, G.; Kanellis, J.; Kavanagh, D.; Pickering, M.C.; Sunder-Plassmann, G.; Walker, P.D.; Wang, Z.; Ahmad, Z.; et al. Efficacy and safety of pegcetacoplan in kidney transplant recipients with recurrent complement 3 glomerulopathy or primary immune complex membranoproliferative glomerulonephritis. *Kidney Int. Rep.* **2025**, *10*, 87–98. [CrossRef]
101. Tarragón, B.; Peleg, Y.; Jagannathan, G.; Sekulic, M.; Chang, J.-H.; Cohen, D.J.; Crew, R.J.; Dube, G.K.; Fernandez, H.E.; Husain, S.A.; et al. C3 glomerulopathy recurs early after kidney transplantation in serial biopsies performed within the first 2 years after transplantation. *Clin. J. Am. Soc. Nephrol.* **2024**, *19*, 1005–1015. [CrossRef]
102. Infante, B.; Rossini, M.; Leo, S.; Troise, D.; Netti, G.S.; Ranieri, E.; Gesualdo, L.; Castellano, G.; Stallone, G. Recurrent glomerulonephritis after renal transplantation: The clinical problem. *Int. J. Mol. Sci.* **2020**, *21*, 5954. [CrossRef]
103. Noris, M.; Remuzzi, G. C3G and Ig-MPGN-treatment standard. *Nephrol. Dial. Transplant.* **2024**, *39*, 202–214. [CrossRef]
104. Coche, S.; Sprangers, B.; Van Laecke, S.; Weekers, L.; De Meyer, V.; Hellemans, R.; Castanares, D.; Ameye, H.; Goffin, E.; Demoulin, N.; et al. Recurrence and outcome of anti-glomerular basement membrane glomerulonephritis after kidney transplantation. *Kidney Int. Rep.* **2021**, *6*, 1888–1894. [CrossRef] [PubMed]
105. Mignano, S.E.; Nasr, S.H.; Fidler, M.E.; Herrera Hernandez, L.P.; Alexander, M.P.; Sethi, S.; Messias, N.; Alhamad, T.; Alrata, L.; Albadri, S.T.; et al. Recurrent atypical antiglomerular basement membrane nephritis in the kidney transplant. *Am. J. Transplant.* **2024**, *24*, 123–133. [CrossRef] [PubMed]
106. Segelmark, M.; Hellmark, T. Anti-glomerular basement membrane disease: An update on subgroups, pathogenesis and therapies. *Nephrol. Dial. Transplant.* **2019**, *34*, 1826–1832. [CrossRef] [PubMed]
107. McAdoo, S.P.; Pusey, C.D. Anti-glomerular basement membrane disease. *Clin. J. Am. Soc. Nephrol.* **2017**, *12*, 1162–1172. [CrossRef] [PubMed]
108. Contreras, G.; Mattiazzi, A.; Guerra, G.; Ortega, L.M.; Tozman, E.C.; Li, H.; Tamariz, L.; Carvalho, C.; Kupin, W.; Ladino, M.; et al. Recurrence of lupus nephritis after kidney transplantation. *J. Am. Soc. Nephrol.* **2010**, *21*, 1200–1207. [CrossRef]
109. Norby, G.E.; Strøm, E.H.; Midtvedt, K.; Hartmann, A.; Gilboe, I.-M.; Leivestad, T.; Stenstrøm, J.; Holdaas, H. Recurrent lupus nephritis after kidney transplantation: A surveillance biopsy study. *Ann. Rheum. Dis.* **2010**, *69*, 1484–1487. [CrossRef]
110. Kidney Disease: Improving Global Outcomes (KDIGO); Lupus Nephritis Work Group. KDIGO 2024 clinical practice guideline for the management of LUPUS NEPHRITIS. *Kidney Int.* **2024**, *105*, S1–S69. [CrossRef]
111. Sammaritano, L.R.; Askanase, A.; Bermas, B.L.; Dall'Era, M.; Duarte-García, A.; Hiraki, L.T.; Rovin, B.H.; Son, M.B.F.; Alvarado, A.; Aranow, C.; et al. 2024 American college of rheumatology (ACR) guideline for the screening, treatment, and management of lupus nephritis. *Arthritis Rheumatol.* **2025**, *77*, 1115–1135. [CrossRef]
112. Albuquerque, B.C.; Salles, V.B.; Tajra RDde, P.; Rodrigues, C.E.M. Outcome and prognosis of patients with lupus nephritis submitted to renal transplantation. *Sci. Rep.* **2019**, *9*, 11611. [CrossRef] [PubMed]
113. Rodelo, J.; González, L.A.; Ustáriz, J.; Matera, S.; Pérez, K.; Ramírez, Z.; Arias, L.F.; García, Á.; Arbeláez, M.; Henao, J. Kidney transplantation outcomes in lupus nephritis: A 37-year single-center experience from Latin America. *Lupus* **2021**, *30*, 1644–1659. [CrossRef]
114. Çeltİk, A.; Şen, S.; Tamer, A.F.; Yılmaz, M.; Sarsık, B.; Özkahya, M.; Başçı, A.; Töz, H. Recurrent lupus nephritis after transplantation: Clinicopathological evaluation with protocol biopsies. *Nephrology* **2016**, *21*, 601–607. [CrossRef]
115. Moroni, G.; Calatroni, M.; Ponticelli, C. The Recurrence of Systemic Diseases in Kidney Transplantation. *J. Clin. Med.* **2025**, *14*, 2592. [CrossRef] [PubMed]
116. Meehan, S.M.; Chang, A.; Khurana, A.; Baliga, R.; Kadambi, P.V.; Javaid, B. Pauci-immune and immune glomerular lesions in kidney transplants for systemic lupus erythematosus. *Clin. J. Am. Soc. Nephrol.* **2008**, *3*, 1469–1478. [CrossRef]
117. Siegel, C.H.; Sammaritano, L.R. Systemic lupus erythematosus: A review. *JAMA* **2024**, *331*, 1480–1491. [CrossRef]
118. Masset, C.; Kandel-Aznar, C.; Dantal, J.; Giral, M.; Hourmant, M.; Blancho, G.; Garandeau, C. Early and late ANCA vasculitis relapses after kidney transplantation may have different presentations. *Clin. Kidney J.* **2022**, *15*, 1021–1023. [CrossRef]
119. Hruskova, Z.; Geetha, D.; Tesar, V. Renal transplantation in anti-neutrophil cytoplasmic antibody-associated vasculitis. *Nephrol. Dial. Transplant.* **2015**, *30* (Suppl. 1), i159–i163. [CrossRef]
120. Lau, D.; Summers, S.; Amos, L.; Simpson, I.; Mulley, W. Recurrence of anti-neutrophil cytoplasmic antibody vasculitis in the kidney allograft. *Nephrology* **2012**, *17* (Suppl. S1), 16–19. [CrossRef]
121. Silva, R.M.; Leal, R.; Marques, M.G.; Rodrigues, L.; Santos, L.; Romãozinho, C.; Alves, R.; Figueiredo, A. Renal transplantation in antineutrophil cytoplasmic antibody-associated vasculitis: A single-center 10-year experience. *Transplant. Proc.* **2023**, *55*, 1396–1399. [CrossRef]
122. Kidney Disease: Improving Global Outcomes (KDIGO); ANCA Vasculitis Work Group. KDIGO 2024 clinical practice guideline for the management of antineutrophil cytoplasmic antibody (ANCA)-associated vasculitis. *Kidney Int.* **2024**, *105*, S71–S116. [CrossRef] [PubMed]

123. Göçeroğlu, A.; Rahmattulla, C.; Berden, A.E.; Reinders, M.E.J.; Wolterbeek, R.; Steenbergen, E.J.; Hilbrands, L.B.; Noorlander, I.; Berger, S.P.; Peutz-Kootstra, C.J.; et al. The Dutch Transplantation in Vasculitis (DUTRAVAS) Study: Outcome of Renal Transplantation in Antineutrophil Cytoplasmic Antibody-associated Glomerulonephritis. *Transplantation* **2016**, *100*, 916–924 [CrossRef] [PubMed]
124. Murakami, C.; Manoharan, P.; Carter-Monroe, N.; Geetha, D. Rituximab for remission induction in recurrent ANCA-associated glomerulonephritis postkidney transplant. *Transpl. Int.* **2013**, *26*, 1225–1231. [CrossRef]
125. Geetha, D.; Seo, P.; Specks, U.; Fervenza, F.C. Successful induction of remission with rituximab for relapse of ANCA-associated vasculitis post-kidney transplant: Report of two cases. *Am. J. Transplant.* **2007**, *7*, 2821–2825. [CrossRef]
126. Gulati, K.; Edwards, H.; Prendecki, M.; Cairns, T.D.; Condon, M.; Galliford, J.; Griffith, M.; Levy, J.B.; Tam, F.W.; Tanna, A.; et al. Combination treatment with rituximab, low-dose cyclophosphamide and plasma exchange for severe antineutrophil cytoplasmic antibody-associated vasculitis. *Kidney Int.* **2021**, *100*, 1316–1324. [CrossRef] [PubMed]

Journal of
Clinical Medicine

MDPI

Article

Selection Patterns and Outcomes of Kidney Transplantation Versus Dialysis in Lung Recipients with End-Stage Renal Disease: A Single-Center Retrospective-Observational Study

Fahim Kanani [1,*], Mordechai R. Kramer [2], Mohamad Atamna [2], Abed Elrahman Dahly [1], Aviad Gravets [1], Wladimir Tennak [1], Sigal Eisner [1] and Eviatar Nesher [1]

[1] Department of Transplantation, Beilinson Medical Centre, Gray Faculty of Medicine, Tel Aviv University, Petah Tiqwa 4941492, Israel; dahle.abed@clalit.org.il (A.E.D.); avuadgr@clalit.org.il (A.G.); wladimirtn@clalilt.org.ol (W.T.); sigalei@clalit.org.il (S.E.); eviatarne@clalit.or.il (E.N.)

[2] Institute of Pulmonary Medicine, Rabin Medical Center, Beilinson Hospital, Gray Faculty of Medicine, Tel Aviv University, Petah Tiqwa 4941492, Israel; mordechai.r.kremer@clalit.org.il (M.R.K.); mohamadat2@clalit.org.il (M.A.)

* Correspondence: kanani.fahim@gmail.com; Tel.: +972-54-344-7147

Abstract: Background: End-stage renal disease (ESRD) affects up to 25% of lung transplant recipients within 10 years. The selection process for kidney transplantation versus dialysis reflects complex clinical decision-making that has not been systematically characterized. **Methods:** This retrospective observational study analyzed all lung transplant recipients who developed ESRD at our center from 2010 to 2024 (n=32), comparing those receiving kidney transplantation (n = 18) versus those remaining on dialysis (n = 14). We developed an exploratory Clinical Selection Score to retrospectively characterize observed selection patterns and calculated E-values to assess robustness to unmeasured confounding. **Results:** Kidney transplant recipients were younger (35.7 ± 12.9 vs. 48.4 ± 14.8 years, p = 0.013) with better selection characteristics quantified by our Clinical Selection Score (4.1 ± 0.8 vs. 1.6 ± 1.1 points, p < 0.001). The score showed excellent discrimination (C-statistic 0.82). Living donors were available for 88.9% of transplanted patients versus 0% of dialysis patients. In our selected cohorts, mortality was 22.2% in kidney transplant recipients vs. 78.6% in dialysis patients (p = 0.002), with median survival of 161.6 vs. 126.6 months (p = 0.021). After adjustment for age, kidney transplantation was observed to be associated with 72% lower mortality risk (HR 0.28, 95% CI 0.09–0.89, p = 0.031), though selection bias limits causal interpretation. The E-value of 6.61 suggests robustness to unmeasured confounding. **Conclusions:** This observational study describes real-world selection patterns and their associated outcomes in lung transplant recipients with ESRD. While carefully selected patients receiving kidney transplantation experienced favorable results, many patients were appropriately managed with dialysis based on medical and non-medical factors. Our analysis provides transparency about selection criteria and outcomes to inform clinical decision-making. Larger multicenter studies are needed to validate these findings and develop prediction tools.

Keywords: kidney after lung transplantation; clinical selection; real-world evidence; transplant outcomes; ESRD

1. Introduction

The landscape of lung transplantation has evolved dramatically over the past decade, with refined surgical techniques and immunosuppressive protocols yielding unprecedented survival rates exceeding 85% at one year and approaching 60% at five years [1,2]. This success, however, has unmasked a sobering reality: the emergence of chronic kidney disease (CKD) as a formidable barrier to long-term graft and patient survival. Indeed, kidney dysfunction now represents the Achilles' heel of modern lung transplantation. A recent meta-analysis found AKI occurs in 52.5% of lung transplant recipients, with 9.3% requiring RRT [3], while ESRD develops in up to 16% by five years and nearly 25% by a decade post-transplant [4–6].

The pathogenesis of post-lung transplant nephropathy involves pre-transplant vulnerability, perioperative insults, and chronic calcineurin inhibitor (CNI) toxicity. A recent meta-analysis demonstrated AKI occurs in 52.5% of lung transplant recipients, with 9.3% requiring RRT [3]. CNI therapy, while essential for preventing rejection, contributes to progressive nephrotoxicity with 21% of patients developing kidney dysfunction [7]. This creates a therapeutic paradox: the immunosuppression preserving lung function simultaneously destroys kidney function [8].

When ESRD inevitably develops—typically 5–7 years post-lung transplant—clinicians confront a critical crossroads: chronic dialysis versus kidney transplantation. The data paint a stark picture. Lung transplant recipients relegated to chronic dialysis face dismal outcomes, with median survival rarely exceeding 24 months and five-year survival hovering around 20% [9]. In contrast, successful kidney transplantation in this population, though technically complex and immunologically nuanced, offers the tantalizing prospect of restored kidney function without additional immunosuppressive burden. Recent multicenter analyses suggest that kidney-after-lung transplantation may confer survival benefits comparable to those observed in the general ESRD population, with hazard ratios for mortality approaching 0.73 compared to dialysis-dependent counterparts [9].

Critical knowledge gaps remain regarding optimal timing for kidney transplantation, the influence of pre-existing immunosuppression on outcomes, and the identification of recipients who would benefit from preemptive transplantation. These gaps impede evidence-based decision-making.

Herein, we present our institutional experience spanning 14 years, systematically characterizing the selection process and outcomes of lung transplant recipients with ESRD who received kidney transplantation versus dialysis. Rather than attempting to prove the superiority of one treatment over another—a question confounded by necessary selection bias—we aim to provide transparency about real-world clinical decision-making and its outcomes. Our goal is to demonstrate the feasibility of excellent outcomes in carefully selected patients while providing a methodological framework for future larger studies.

2. Methods

2.1. Study Design and Setting

This retrospective cohort study analysed data from a prospectively maintained transplant registry of a referral center serving as the primary lung transplant facility for a population of 9.5 million (IRB approval: BMC 0525-25). Our institution performs approximately 25–30 lung transplants and 200 living and deceased kidneys annually, with integrated nephrology services facilitating seamless transition to renal replacement therapy when required. This study adhered to the Strengthening the Reporting of Observational Studies in Epidemiology (STROBE) guidelines [10].

2.2. Patient Identification and Selection

From 600 consecutive adult lung transplant recipients (January 2010–December 2024), we identified 32 who progressed to ESRD requiring RRT through systematic screening of our transplant registry, dialysis records, and laboratory surveillance systems. Detailed screening methodology is provided in Supplementary Methods. Inclusion criteria: adult lung transplant recipients (≥18 years) who developed ESRD requiring RRT for >90 days. Exclusion criteria: combined heart-lung transplants, pediatric recipients, and those with <90 days of follow-up after ESRD diagnosis. Scheme 1 shows the COSNSORT diagram for the patient selection flowchart.

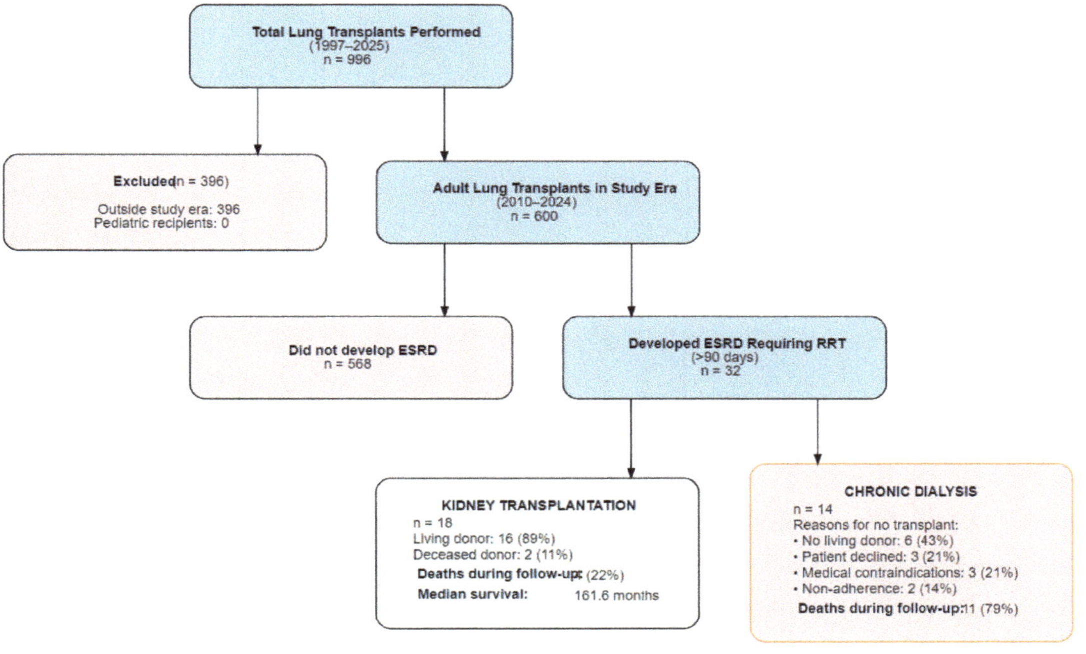

Scheme 1. COSNSORT diagram for the patient selection.

2.3. Definitions

Acute kidney injury (AKI) after lung transplant, followed KDIGO criteria: serum creatinine increase ≥ 0.3 mg/dL within 48 h or ≥1.5 times baseline within 7 days [11]. Chronic kidney disease (CKD) requires an eGFR of <60 mL/min/1.73 m^2 persisting beyond 3 months. ESRD was defined as an eGFR of <15 mL/min/1.73 m^2 or chronic dialysis requirement exceeding 90 days.

2.4. Clinical Decision-Making for RRT Modality

The choice between kidney transplantation and dialysis resulted from a complex interplay of medical criteria, patient preferences, and resource availability. While institutional protocols guided evaluation, final treatment allocation reflected multiple factors:

Medical Criteria:

- Cardiopulmonary reserve (FEV1 >40% predicted, recommended, but not absolute)
- Absence of active malignancy or untreated infection
- Life expectancy considerations
- Non-Medical Determinants:
- Living donor availability (most critical factor)
- Patient preference regarding additional surgery
- Concerns about cumulative surgical risk
- Limited outcome data to guide informed consent
- Geographic/social factors affecting follow-up capability

Notably, some patients with adequate medical criteria declined transplant evaluation due to surgical fatigue or uncertainty about benefits, while others were excluded primarily due to lack of donor availability despite reasonable medical status. This real-world allocation process, rather than strict protocol-driven selection, created comparison groups that reflect clinical practice complexity.

2.5. Clinical Selection Framework

To characterize this selection process retrospectively, we developed an exploratory "Clinical Selection Score" as an exploratory, hypothesis-generating tool—not for clinical use—to quantify observed selection patterns. This score was not used prospectively for treatment decisions but rather calculated post-hoc to understand allocation patterns. The score incorporated five factors based on established prognostic factors in transplant literature:

- Age at ESRD diagnosis (<40 years = 1 point), as age > 60 predicts mortality (HR 1.82, 95% CI 1.34–2.47) [5];
- Lung allograft function (FEV1 > 60% = 1 point), a key selection criterion for subsequent transplantation [9];
- Time from lung transplant to ESRD (>5 years = 1 point), as each dialysis year increases mortality by 6.8% [12];
- Living donor availability (yes = 1 point), associated with superior outcomes in registry data [13];
- Performance status (fully ambulatory = 1 point), identified as prognostic in ISHLT analyses [1].

This 0–5 point score was calculated retrospectively to quantify selection patterns, not to guide treatment. This score requires external validation before any clinical application and is presented solely to provide transparency about selection patterns observed in our cohort.

2.6. Outcomes

The primary outcome was overall survival from lung transplantation. Secondary endpoints included time from lung transplant to ESRD, time from ESRD to RRT initiation, kidney allograft function (eGFR at 1 and 5 years), dialysis dependency at 1 and 3 years, and cause of death.

2.7. Data Collection and Quality Assurance

Data were extracted independently by two researchers using standardized forms. Primary outcome (survival) achieved 100% completeness through national death registry linkage. Time-to-event variables had <5% missingness. Variables with >10% missingness were excluded to avoid imputation bias. For variables with <10% missingness, we used complete case analysis for primary outcomes and multiple imputation for sensitivity analyses.

2.8. Follow-Up Protocol

Follow-up included regular clinical and laboratory assessments per institutional protocols (detailed in Supplementary Methods). Data collection concluded 31 December 2023. No patients were lost to follow-up for the primary outcome.

2.9. Statistical Analysis

Analyses were performed using R version 4.3.0. Continuous variables were expressed as mean $\pm$ standard deviation or median (interquartile range). Categorical variables were presented as frequencies and percentages.

We performed descriptive statistics, Kaplan–Meier survival analysis with log-rank test, and Cox proportional hazards regression. Propensity score matching was attempted but failed due to non-overlapping distributions between groups, confirming the strong selection bias and fundamentally different patient populations that preclude causal inference [14].

For survival analysis, univariate Cox regression identified potential predictors. Variables with $p < 0.10$ were considered for multivariable analysis. Given our sample size of 32 patients with 15 events, we limited multivariable models to 2 covariates following established guidelines. We selected age for adjustment based on its clinical importance and significant univariate association.

Statistical significance was defined as $p < 0.05$. The wide confidence intervals observed (HR 0.28, 95% CI 0.09–0.89) reflect the limited precision inherent to this sample size. All sensitivity analyses, including E-value calculations, competing risks models, and landmark analyses, are presented in Supplementary Materials.

2.10. AI Tool Declaration

The authors used Grammarly and Microsoft Copilot solely for grammar correction and readability enhancement. All scientific content and intellectual contributions remain the exclusive work of the authors.

3. Results

3.1. Patient Characteristics

Of 600 lung transplants (2010–2024), 32 patients (5.3%) developed ESRD: 18 received kidney transplants, 14 remained on dialysis. Kidney recipients were younger (35.7 ± 12.9 vs. 48.4 ± 14.8 years, $p = 0.013$) (Table 1). Primary diagnoses: cystic fibrosis (31.3%), idiopathic pulmonary fibrosis (18.8%). Reasons for non-transplantation: no living donors (43%), patient refusal (21%), medical contraindications (21%), and non-adherence (14%) (Figure 1).

Table 1. Baseline demographics and comorbidities.

Variable	Total ($n = 32$)	Dialysis ($n = 14$)	Kidney Transplant ($n = 18$)	p-Value
Demographics				
Age at lung transplant (years), mean ± SD	41.3 ± 14.9	48.4 ± 14.8	35.7 ± 12.9	0.013
Male sex, n (%)	18 (56.3)	6 (42.9)	10 (55.6)	0.476
BMI (kg/m^2), mean ± SD	27.5 ± 2.8	27.1 ± 2.1	27.9 ± 3.2	0.428
Ethnicity, n (%)				0.812
-Caucasian	24 (75.0)	10 (71.4)	14 (77.8)	
-Other	8 (25.0)	4 (28.6)	4 (22.2)	
Smoking history, n (%)	9 (28.1)	5 (35.7)	4 (22.2)	0.400
Previous abdominal surgery, n (%)	7 (21.9)	3 (21.4)	4 (22.2)	0.957
CMV IgG positive, n (%)	20 (62.5)	9 (64.3)	11 (61.1)	0.854
Primary Pulmonary Diagnosis, n (%)				0.825
-Cystic Fibrosis	10 (31.3)	4 (28.6)	6 (33.3)	
-Idiopathic Pulmonary Fibrosis	6 (18.8)	3 (21.4)	3 (16.7)	
-Emphysema/COPD	4 (12.5)	2 (14.3)	2 (11.1)	
-Other	12 (37.5)	5 (35.7)	7 (38.9)	

Baseline demographics and comorbidities. Comparison of demographic characteristics and pre-transplant comorbidities between lung transplant recipients who developed ESRD and subsequently received kidney transplantation ($n = 18$) versus those maintained on chronic dialysis ($n = 14$). p-values calculated using t-test for continuous variables and chi-square test for categorical variables.

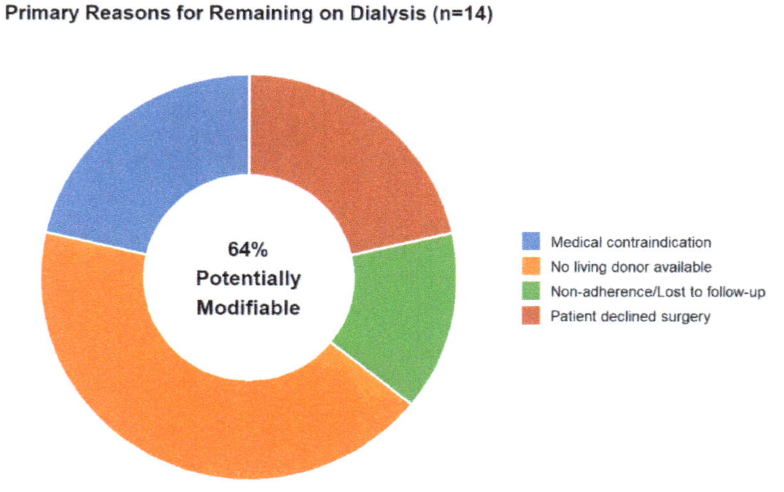

Figure 1. Primary reasons for remaining on dialysis in lung transplant recipients with ESRD (n = 14). Potentially modifiable factors accounted for 64% of cases.

3.2. Transplant Characteristics and Timing

Pre-lung transplant kidney function was similar between groups (eGFR 95.3 ± 30.0 mL/min/1.73 m^2). Median time to ESRD was 5.6 years (IQR 3.8–6.8). Among kidney recipients, 88.9% received living donor organs with minimal cold ischemia (1.47 ± 1.39 h) (Tables 2 and 3).

Table 2. Transplant characteristics and outcomes.

Variable	Total (*n* = 32)	Dialysis (*n* = 14)	Kidney Transplant (*n* = 18)	*p*-Value
Pre-Lung Transplant kidney Function				
eGFR (mL/min/1.73 m^2), mean ± SD	95.3 ± 30.0	91.6 ± 29.8	98.1 ± 30.4	0.548
Serum creatinine (mg/dL), mean ± SD	0.83 ± 0.35	0.87 ± 0.29	0.80 ± 0.39	0.574
Lung Transplant Details				
Type of lung transplant, *n* (%)				0.577
-Single lung	10 (31.3)	6 (42.9)	4 (22.2)	
-Double lung	22 (68.8)	8 (57.1)	14 (77.8)	
Cold ischemia time (hours), mean ± SD	3.2 ± 0.8	3.2 ± 0.7	3.2 ± 0.9	0.990
Perioperative Outcomes				
ICU stay (days), median (IQR)	2 (2–3)	2 (2–6)	2 (2–3)	0.745
Hospital stay (days), median (IQR)	17 (13–24)	16 (12–24)	18 (14–24)	0.421
Early Complications				
AKI after lung transplant, *n* (%)	25 (78.1)	11 (78.6)	14 (77.8)	0.957
Acute Tubular Necrosis (ATN)		9 (81)	11(78.6)	
Primary graft dysfunction grade ≥2, *n* (%)	7 (21.9)	4 (28.6)	3 (16.7)	0.421
Reintubation, *n* (%)	2 (6.3)	1 (7.1)	1 (5.6)	0.856
Early postoperative dialysis, *n* (%)	2 (6.3)	1 (7.1)	1 (5.6)	0.856
Progression to ESRD				
Time from lung to ESRD (years), median (IQR)	5.6 (3.8–6.8)	5.4 (2.2–6.8)	5.9 (3.9–7.1)	0.556
Kidney Transplant Characteristics				
Time from ESRD to kidney transplant (years), median (IQR)	-	N/A	0.5 (0.3–1.9)	-
Time from lung to kidney transplant (years), median (IQR)	-	N/A	6.8 (5.5–9.1)	-
Time on dialysis before kidney transplant (months), median (IQR) *	-	N/A	1.4 (0.2–5.0)	-
Donor type, *n* (%)				
-Living donor	-	N/A	16 (88.9)	-
-Deceased donor	-	N/A	2 (11.1)	-
Cold ischemia time kidney (hours), mean ± SD	-	N/A	1.47 ± 1.39	-
Operative time kidney (minutes), mean ± SD	-	N/A	205 ± 34.8	-
Hospital stay kidney transplant (days), median (IQR)	-	N/A	8 (8–10)	-

* For non-preemptive transplants only (*n* = 16). Lung transplant operative details, perioperative outcomes, and kidney transplant-specific characteristics. Data presented for the total cohort and stratified by ultimate renal replacement therapy modality. AKI = acute kidney injury, defined by KDIGO criteria. N/A = not applicable for dialysis group. Note: The combined lung-kidney transplant data (*n* = 2) can be mentioned in the text rather than the table to avoid complexity.

Table 3. Kidney transplant-specific characteristics ($n = 18$).

Variable	Kidney Transplant Recipients ($n = 18$)
Timing Variables	
Time from ESRD to kidney transplant (years), median (IQR)	0.5 (0.3–1.9)
Time from lung to kidney transplant (years), median (IQR)	6.8 (5.5–9.1)
Time from ESRD diagnosis to dialysis initiation (months), median (IQR)	0.35 (0.0–3.9)
Time on dialysis before kidney transplant (months), median (IQR) *	1.4 (0.2–5.0)
Donor and Surgical Characteristics	
Donor type, n (%)	
-Living donor	16 (88.9)
-Deceased donor	2 (11.1)
Cold ischemia time kidney (hours), mean ± SD	1.47 ± 1.39
Operative time kidney (minutes), mean ± SD	205 ± 34.8
Hospital stay kidney transplant (days), median (IQR)	8 (8–10)
Combined Transplants	
Combined lung-kidney transplant, n (%)	2 (11.1)
Total operative time for combined (minutes)	485 ± 78
ICU stay for combined cases (days)	7 (6–8)
Hospital stay for combined cases (days)	22 (18–26)

* For non-preemptive transplants only ($n = 16$).

3.3. Clinical Selection Patterns

The exploratory Clinical Selection Score demonstrated discrimination in our cohort (C-statistic 0.82, 95% CI 0.71–0.93) with kidney transplant recipients having higher scores (4.1 ± 0.8 vs. 1.6 ± 1.1, $p < 0.001$). Bootstrap validation (1000 iterations) yielded a corrected C-statistic of 0.79 (95% CI 0.68–0.90), suggesting modest optimism but reasonable internal consistency. Key selection factors included age < 40 years (72.2% vs. 21.4%, $p = 0.004$), FEV1 > 60% (66.7% vs. 28.6%, $p = 0.033$), and living donor availability (88.9% vs. 0%, $p < 0.001$) (Table S9).

3.4. Long-Term Outcomes

All kidney recipients achieved immediate graft function (eGFR 74.9 ± 26.2 mL/min/1.73 m^2 at 1 year). Mortality was 22.2% in kidney recipients vs. 78.6% in dialysis patients ($p = 0.002$), with median survival 161.6 vs. 126.6 months ($p = 0.021$) (Table 4, Figure 2).

Table 4. Long-term outcomes and follow-up.

Variable	Total ($n = 32$)	Dialysis ($n = 14$)	Kidney Transplant ($n = 18$)	p-Value
kidney Replacement Outcomes				
Dialysis dependency at 1 year, n (%) *	16 (66.7)	14 (100)	2 (11.1)	<0.001
Dialysis dependency at 3 years, n (%) **	15 (93.8)	14 (100)	1 (5.6)	<0.001
Kidney Graft Function ($n = 18$)				
Immediate graft function, n (%)	-	-	18 (100)	
Delayed graft function, n (%)	-	-	0 (0)	
Rejection episodes, n (%)	-	-	3 (16.7)	
eGFR at 1 year (mL/min/1.73 m^2), mean ± SD ***	-	-	74.9 ± 26.2	
eGFR at 5 years (mL/min/1.73 m^2), mean ± SD ****	-	-	57.0 ± 39.4	
Survival Outcomes				
Deaths during follow-up, n (%)	15 (46.9)	11 (78.6)	4 (22.2)	0.002
Median survival from lung transplant (months)	133.5	126.6	161.6	0.021
Cause of Death, n (%) ****				0.198
-Infection/Sepsis	8 (53.3)	7 (63.6)	1 (25.0)	
-Lung rejection	1 (6.7)	1 (9.1)	0 (0)	
-Other/Unknown	6 (40.0)	3 (27.3)	3 (75.0)	

* $n = 24$ patients evaluable at 1 year; ** $n = 16$ patients evaluable at 3 years; *** $n = 17$ patients with available data; **** $n = 5$ patients with available data; Total deaths $n = 15$. Renal replacement therapy outcomes, kidney graft function parameters, and mortality data stratified by treatment group. Denominators vary due to differential follow-up times and data availability, as noted.

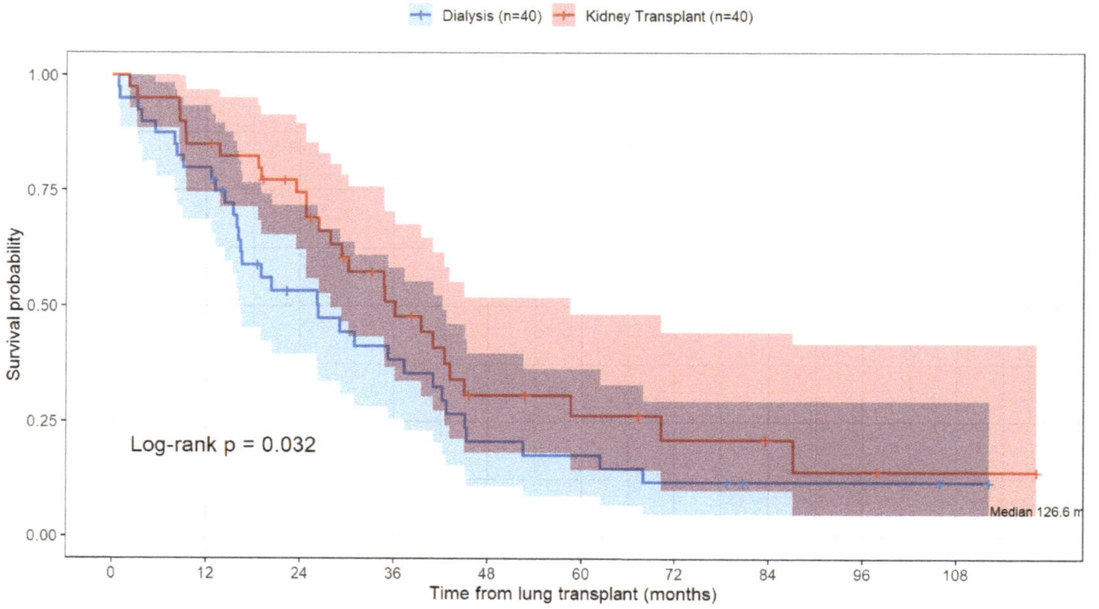

Figure 2. Overall survival from lung transplantation comparing kidney transplant recipients versus dialysis patients. Kaplan–Meier survival curves comparing patients who received kidney transplantation (n = 18, red) versus those maintained on dialysis (n = 14, blue) from the time of lung transplantation. Shaded areas represent 95% confidence intervals. Log-rank p = 0.032. Median survival: kidney transplant 161.6 months, dialysis 126.6 months.

3.5. Survival Analysis

Overall mortality was 22.2% in kidney transplant recipients versus 78.6% in dialysis patients (p = 0.002), with median survival of 161.6 versus 126.6 months (log-rank p = 0.032) (Figure 2, Table 5). Multivariate Cox regression showed kidney transplantation was associated with 72% lower mortality risk (HR 0.28, 95% CI 0.09–0.89, p = 0.031) Figure 3 after adjusting for age Table 6 (Table S7). Propensity matching failed due to non-overlapping distributions.

Table 5. Univariate Cox regression analysis for mortality.

Variable	HR (95% CI)	p-Value
Kidney transplant (vs. dialysis) *	0.24 (0.08–0.75)	0.014
Age at lung transplant (per year) *	1.03 (1.00–1.06)	0.048
Male sex	0.68 (0.25–1.85)	0.449
Body Mass Index (per unit)	1.05 (0.91–1.21)	0.514
Smoking history	1.48 (0.53–4.13)	0.454
Time from lung to ESRD (per year)	0.98 (0.88–1.10)	0.754
AKI after lung transplant	1.19 (0.34–4.19)	0.786
Primary graft dysfunction grade ≥ 2	0.93 (0.26–3.28)	0.910
Early postoperative dialysis	0.64 (0.08–4.82)	0.663

Univariate Cox regression analysis for mortality hazard ratios for all-cause mortality from lung transplantation.
* Variables with $p < 0.10$ were considered for multivariable analysis.

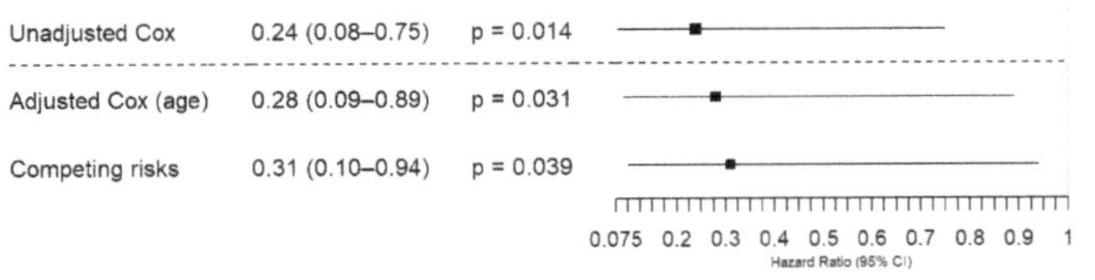

Figure 3. Hazard ratios for mortality comparing kidney transplantation versus dialysis. Forest plot showing hazard ratios (95% CI) from different analytical approaches: unadjusted Cox regression (HR 0.24, 95% CI 0.08–0.75, $p = 0.014$), age-adjusted Cox regression (HR 0.28, 95% CI 0.09–0.89, $p = 0.031$), and competing risks analysis (HR 0.31, 95% CI 0.10–0.94, $p = 0.039$).

Table 6. Multivariate Cox regression analysis for mortality.

Variable	HR (95% CI)	*p*-Value
Kidney transplant (vs. dialysis) *	0.28 (0.09–0.89)	0.031
Age at lung transplant (per year) *	1.03 (1.00–1.06)	0.062

Multivariate Cox regression analysis for mortality: Age-adjusted hazard ratio for mortality comparing kidney transplantation versus dialysis. Model limited to two covariates based on sample size constraints (15 events). * Variables with $p < 0.10$ in univariate analysis were included in the multivariate model.

3.6. Sensitivity Analyses

The E-value of 6.61 indicated robust findings unlikely to be explained by unmeasured confounding. Competing risk analysis confirmed the benefit (subdistribution HR 0.31, 95% CI 0.10–0.94, $p = 0.039$). Landmark analysis at 6 months, addressing immortal time bias, demonstrated continued survival differences beyond the early post-transplant period (Figures 2 and 3). Propensity matching failed due to non-overlap, with zero deaths in the matched cohort of 12 patients.

Distribution of reasons why lung transplant recipients with ESRD remained on chronic dialysis. Medical contraindications (21%, $n = 3$) included active malignancy, severe cardiopulmonary disease, or active infection. Potentially modifiable barriers (64%, $n = 9$) comprised: no living donor available (43%, $n = 6$), patient declined surgery (21%, $n = 3$), and non-adherence/lost to follow-up (14%, $n = 2$) (Figure 1).

4. Discussion

Our investigation of 32 lung transplant recipients with ESRD over 14 years provides insights into real-world clinical selection patterns and their associated outcomes. Our relatively low ESRD incidence (5.3%) compared to 7.6% in the ISHLT registry [15] may reflect our center's CNI minimization protocols and early nephrology engagement. The primary observation—kidney transplant recipients experienced 72% lower mortality risk (HR 0.28, 95% CI 0.09–0.89)—should be interpreted as reflecting successful patient selection rather than demonstrating treatment superiority. These associations primarily represent the outcomes of selecting younger, healthier candidates with available living donors, not evidence of causal benefit. While we cannot separate selection effects from potential treatment effects in this observational analysis, quantifying these selection patterns provides transparency about real-world clinical decision-making

4.1. The Selection Reality

Our Clinical Selection Score achieved efficient discrimination (C-statistic 0.82) using simple, clinically intuitive variables. The stark differences between groups—younger age (35.7 vs. 48.4 years), living donor availability (89% vs. 0%), and preserved lung function—reflect real-world selection patterns that have evolved through clinical experience. The significance of age aligns with Ruebner et al.'s retrospective multicenter cohort study [5], identifying age >60 as an independent mortality predictor (HR 1.82, 95% CI 1.34–2.47). These findings parallel larger studies showing similar selection criteria [9], though our 89% living donor rate substantially exceeds the 30% national average [13], suggesting unique institutional or population characteristics.

Our analysis reveals that 64% of dialysis patients faced modifiable barriers (lack of donors or patient preference) rather than medical contraindications, representing opportunities for intervention rather than inevitable outcomes.

4.2. The Pathophysiology of Progression

The high incidence of AKI (78.1%) in our cohort aligns with the 52.5% rate reported in recent meta-analyses [3], highlighting the vulnerability of lung transplant recipients to renal injury. While we did not systematically classify AKI etiologies, the literature suggests ischemic ATN from perioperative hemodynamic instability represents the predominant cause, accounting for approximately 55–60% of cases.

The progression from AKI to ESRD appears multifactorial. Beyond the initial insult, ongoing CNI exposure likely plays a critical role. The Cochrane review [7] demonstrated that 21% of lung transplant recipients develop kidney dysfunction on CNI therapy, with our cohort's median 5.6-year progression to ESRD suggesting cumulative nephrotoxic effects. This creates a therapeutic dilemma: the immunosuppression preserving lung function simultaneously deteriorates kidney function, ultimately necessitating the very decision our study examines—dialysis versus kidney transplantation.

4.3. Temporal Dynamics: The Critical Window

The median interval from ESRD to kidney transplantation—six months—represents a critical finding. This remarkably short duration contrasts sharply with the general ESRD population's median wait time exceeding 3.6 years [16], reflecting both urgency recognition and 89% living donation. Weinhandl et al. [12] demonstrated that each year on dialysis increases post-transplant mortality by 6.8%. The brief pre-transplant dialysis exposure in our transplanted patients may have contributed to the favorable outcomes observed. Supporting preemptive transplantation, Kasiske et al. showed 23% lower mortality when transplantation occurs before dialysis [17].

4.4. Interpreting the Outcomes

The observed survival differences require cautious interpretation. These associations do not establish causality, and the favorable outcomes in kidney transplant recipients likely reflect both our selection of healthier candidates and any potential treatment benefits. Our exploratory analysis cannot distinguish between these effects. The true treatment benefit, if any, is likely substantially smaller than the 72% risk reduction observed.

The outcomes in both groups suggest appropriate patient management. The 78% 5-year survival in kidney transplant recipients demonstrates outcomes achievable with careful selection, while the 21% 5-year survival in dialysis patients aligns with registry data showing 20–30% 5-year survival in dialysis-dependent lung recipients [1].

4.5. Mortality Patterns

The predominance of infectious deaths in dialysis patients (63.6% vs. 25%) likely reflects the combined burden of immunosuppression and uremia. The higher proportion of 'other/unknown' causes in transplant recipients (75% vs. 27.3%) warrants careful interpretation. While we lack cardiac-specific mortality data, international registry data indicate cardiovascular death accounts for 15–20% of mortality in lung transplant recipients [1]. Our substantial 'other/unknown' category may encompass such cardiovascular events, though this remains speculative without systematic adjudication. Importantly, these ostensibly favorable outcomes in transplant recipients may primarily reflect our selection of candidates with optimal prognostic features rather than demonstrating the therapeutic superiority of kidney transplantation.

4.6. Immunological Advantages

The pre-existing immunosuppressed state creates unique advantages for subsequent kidney transplantation. Our 17% rejection rate compares favorably to 35–40% in de novo kidney transplants [13]. Kovacs et al. recently demonstrated that lung transplant recipients exhibit persistent donor-specific hyporesponsiveness, with reduced frequencies of donor-reactive T cells (0.8% vs. 2.4% in controls, $p < 0.001$) [18]. This acquired tolerance may facilitate kidney engraftment and contribute to the excellent outcomes observed.

4.7. Clinical Framework

Our exploratory analysis identified potential clinical phenotypes based on observed selection patterns. While these groupings showed different outcomes in our cohort (score 4–5: 82% 5-year survival; score 2–3: 54%; score 0–1: 25%), this framework is hypothesis-generating and requires prospective validation before clinical application. The score serves primarily to make transparent the factors that influenced real-world treatment allocation in our center.

4.8. Strengths and Limitations

Our study has several important limitations. The primary limitation is our sample size of 32 patients with 15 deaths, which constrains statistical power to detect modest effect sizes and limits multivariable modeling to essential covariates. The wide confidence intervals reflect this imprecision, and the inability to perform successful propensity matching further illustrates these constraints. While we achieved adequate power for the large observed effect (72% risk reduction), smaller but clinically meaningful differences may have been missed. Moreover, the limited sample size not only constrains statistical power but also results in wide confidence intervals (HR 0.09–0.89), reducing the precision of our effect estimates. This constraint precluded more comprehensive multivariable modeling, leaving the possibility of residual confounding despite adjustment for key covariates. Most importantly, this selection bias is not merely a limitation but the primary driver of our findings. The observed associations should be interpreted as descriptive of our selection process rather than evidence of treatment benefit. Second, the single-center design limits generalizability, particularly given our exceptionally high living donor rate (89% vs. 30% nationally), which may reflect unique institutional or population characteristics. These findings reflect our specific institutional patterns and should not be generalized to other centers without validation. Our results describe a single-center experience and may not apply to institutions with different donor availability or selection practices. Third, the Clinical Selection Score, while demonstrating good discrimination, lacks external validation and should be considered exploratory. Fourth, we did not collect data on cardiovascular medications, diabetes management, or antiplatelet therapy, which may differ between groups and influence outcomes. Future studies should examine whether optimized medical management contributes to the survival benefit observed in transplant recipients. Finally, as with all observational studies, unmeasured confounding remains possible despite our robust E-value analysis.

5. Conclusions

In conclusion, our single-center observational study describes selection patterns and associated outcomes in lung transplant recipients with ESRD. The observed differences between the kidney transplant and dialysis groups primarily reflect selection practices rather than treatment effects. While carefully selected patients achieved favorable outcomes with kidney transplantation, many patients were appropriately managed with dialysis based on individual circumstances. These descriptive findings provide transparency about real-world decision-making but cannot establish optimal treatment strategies. Future multicenter studies with adequate power are needed to develop and validate predictive tools for this complex patient population.

Supplementary Materials: The following supporting information can be downloaded at: https://www.mdpi.com/article/10.3390/jcm14197017/s1. Figure S1: Overview of Lung Transplant Program Outcomes (1997–2025); Figure S2. Primary Pulmonary Diagnoses Leading to Lung Transplantation; Figure S3. Long-term Survival Following Lung Transplantation; Figure S4. Overview of Lung Transplant Program Outcomes (1997–2025); Table S1: Complete Statistical Analysis Summary; Table S2: Time Interval Analysis—Impact on Mortality; Table S3: Patient Flow and Timing; Table S4: Subgroup Analysis by Timing of Kidney Transplant; Table S5: Causes of Death by Treatment Group; Table S6: Model Diagnostics; Table S7: Sample Size Calculation for Future Studies. Tables S8–S10: These tables present exploratory, hypothesis-generating findings from a small single-center cohort that should not guide clinical practice but highlight patterns requiring validation in larger multicenter studies Table S8: Number Needed to Treat (NNT) Analysis; Table S9: Clinical Selection Score Components and Their Association with Treatment Allocation; Table S10: Clinical Phenotypes and Outcomes. References [19,20] are cited in the supplementary materials.

Author Contributions: Conceptualization, F.K. and E.N.; methodology, F.K.; software, A.G.; validation, F.K., M.R.K. and E.N.; formal analysis, F.K. and A.G.; investigation, F.K., A.E.D., W.T. and S.E.; resources, M.A. and M.R.K.; data curation, M.A. and A.G.; writing—original draft preparation, F.K.; writing—review and editing, F.K., M.A., A.E.D., A.G., W.T., M.R.K., S.E. and E.N.; visualization, F.K. and A.G.; supervision, M.R.K. and E.N.; project administration, F.K. and E.N.; funding acquisition, E.N. All authors have read and agreed to the published version of the manuscript.

Funding: This research received no external funding.

Institutional Review Board Statement: This study was approved by the Boston Medical Center Institutional Review Board (IRB approval: RMC 0804-23, Initial Approval Date: 5 December 2023, Extension Approval: Granted on 21 January 2025, valid until 21 January 2026).

Informed Consent Statement: The requirement for individual consent was waived due to the retrospective nature of the study.

Data Availability Statement: The datasets used and/or analyzed during the current study are available from the corresponding author on reasonable request.

Acknowledgments: The authors used at the time of writing, Grammarly (version 14.1255.0, and GitHub Copilot version 1.7.4421) solely for grammar correction and readability enhancement. All scientific content and intellectual contributions remain the exclusive work of the authors.

Conflicts of Interest: The authors declare no conflict of interests.

Abbreviations

AKI:	Acute kidney injury
BMI:	Body mass index
CI:	Confidence interval
CKD:	Chronic kidney disease
CKD-EPI:	Chronic Kidney Disease Epidemiology Collaboration
CLAD:	Chronic lung allograft dysfunction
CMV:	Cytomegalovirus
CNI:	Calcineurin inhibitor

COPD:	Chronic obstructive pulmonary disease
eGFR:	Estimated glomerular filtration rate
EHR:	Electronic health record
ESRD:	End-stage renal disease
FEV1:	Forced expiratory volume in 1 s
HR:	Hazard ratio
ICD-10:	International Classification of Diseases, 10th Revision
ICU:	Intensive care unit
IPW:	Inverse probability weighting
IQR:	Interquartile range
IRB:	Institutional Review Board
ISHLT:	International Society for Heart and Lung Transplantation
KDIGO:	Kidney Disease: Improving Global Outcomes
NNT:	Number needed to treat
OPTN:	Organ Procurement and Transplantation Network
PSM:	Propensity score matching
RMST:	Restricted mean survival time
RRT:	Renal replacement therapy
SD:	Standard deviation
SMD:	Standardized mean difference
SRTR:	Scientific Registry of Transplant Recipients

References

1. Khush, K.K.; Hsich, E.; Potena, L.; Cherikh, W.S.; Chambers, D.C.; Harhay, M.O.; Hayes, D.; Perch, M.; Sadavarte, A.; Toll, A.; et al. The International Thoracic Organ Transplant Registry of the International Society for Heart and Lung Transplantation: Thirty-eighth adult heart transplantation report—2021; Focus on recipient characteristics. *J. Heart Lung Transplant.* **2021**, *40*, 1035–1049. [CrossRef] [PubMed]
2. Yusen, R.D.; Edwards, L.B.; Dipchand, A.I.; Goldfarb, S.B.; Kucheryavaya, A.Y.; Levvey, B.J.; Lund, L.H.; Meiser, B.; Rossano, J.W.; Stehlik, J. The Registry of the International Society for Heart and Lung Transplantation: Thirty-third Adult Lung and Heart–Lung Transplant Report—2016; Focus Theme: Primary Diagnostic Indications for Transplant. *J. Heart Lung Transplant.* **2016**, *35*, 1170–1184. [CrossRef] [PubMed]
3. Lertjitbanjong, P.; Thongprayoon, C.; Cheungpasitporn, W.; O'corragain, O.A.; Srivali, N.; Bathini, T.; Watthanasuntorn, K.; Aeddula, N.R.; Salim, S.A.; Ungprasert, P.; et al. Acute Kidney Injury after Lung Transplantation: A Systematic Review and Meta-Analysis. *J. Clin. Med.* **2019**, *8*, 1713. [CrossRef] [PubMed]
4. Bloom, R.; Doyle, A. Kidney Disease After Heart and Lung Transplantation. *Am. J. Transplant.* **2006**, *6*, 671–679. [CrossRef] [PubMed]
5. Ruebner, R.L.; Reese, P.P.; Denburg, M.R.; Abt, P.L.; Furth, S.L. End-Stage Kidney Disease After Pediatric Nonrenal Solid Organ Transplantation. *Pediatrics* **2013**, *132*, e1319–e1326. [CrossRef] [PubMed]
6. Cosgun, T.; Tomaszek, S.; Opitz, I.; Wilhelm, M.; Schuurmans, M.M.; Weder, W.; Inci, I. Single-center experience with intra-operative extracorporeal membrane oxygenation use in lung transplantation. *Int. J. Artif. Organs* **2017**, *41*, 89–93. [CrossRef] [PubMed]
7. Penninga, L.; Møller, C.H.; Penninga, E.I.; Iversen, M.; Gluud, C.; Steinbrüchel, D.A. Antibody induction therapy for lung transplant recipients. *Cochrane Database Syst. Rev.* **2013**, *2013*, CD008927. [CrossRef] [PubMed]
8. Jing, L.; Chen, W.; Guo, L.; Zhao, L.; Liang, C.; Chen, J.; Wang, C. Acute kidney injury after lung transplantation: A narrative review. *Ann. Transl. Med.* **2021**, *9*, 717. [CrossRef] [PubMed]
9. Osho, A.A.; Hirji, S.A.; Castleberry, A.W.; Mulvihill, M.S.; Ganapathi, A.M.; Speicher, P.J.; Yerokun, B.; Snyder, L.D.; Davis, R.D.; Hartwig, M.G. Long-term survival following kidney transplantation in previous lung transplant recipients-An analysis of the unos registry. *Clin. Transplant.* **2017**, *31*, e12953. [CrossRef] [PubMed]
10. Von Elm, E.; Altman, D.G.; Egger, M.; Pocock, S.J.; Gøtzsche, P.C.; Vandenbroucke, J.P. The Strengthening the Reporting of Observational Studies in Epidemiology (STROBE) statement: Guidelines for reporting observational studies. *J. Clin. Epidemiol.* **2008**, *61*, 344–349. [CrossRef] [PubMed]
11. Stevens, P.E.; Ahmed, S.B.; Carrero, J.J.; Foster, B.; Francis, A.; Hall, R.K.; Herrington, W.G.; Hill, G.; Inker, L.A.; Kazancıoğlu, R.; et al. KDIGO 2024 Clinical Practice Guideline for the Evaluation and Management of Chronic Kidney Disease. *Kidney Int.* **2024**, *105*, S117–S314. [CrossRef] [PubMed]

12. Weinhandl, E.D.; Gilbertson, D.T.; Collins, A.J. Mortality, Hospitalization, and Technique Failure in Daily Home Hemodialysis and Matched Peritoneal Dialysis Patients: A Matched Cohort Study. *Am. J. Kidney Dis.* **2016**, *67*, 98–110. [CrossRef] [PubMed]
13. Organ Procurement and Transplantation Network/Scientific Registry of Transplant Recipients. OPTN/SRTR 2023 Annual Report. Available online: https://srtr.transplant.hrsa.gov/ADR/Chapter?name=Kidney&year=2023 (accessed on 1 March 2024).
14. Stuart, E.A.; Lee, B.K.; Leacy, F.P. Prognostic score–based balance measures can be a useful diagnostic for propensity score methods in comparative effectiveness research. *J. Clin. Epidemiol.* **2013**, *66*, S84–S90.e1. [CrossRef] [PubMed]
15. Singh, T.P.; Cherikh, W.S.; Hsich, E.; Harhay, M.O.; Hayes, D.; Perch, M.; Potena, L.; Sadavarte, A.; Zuckermann, A.; Stehlik, J. The International thoracic organ transplant registry of the international society for heart and lung transplantation: Twenty-fifth pediatric heart transplantation report—2022; focus on infant heart transplantation. *J. Heart Lung Transplant.* **2022**, *41*, 1357–1365. [CrossRef] [PubMed]
16. Lentine, K.L.; Smith, J.M.; Lyden, G.R.; Miller, J.M.; Dolan, T.G.; Bradbrook, K.; Larkin, L.; Temple, K.; Handarova, D.K.; Weiss, S.; et al. OPTN/SRTR 2022 Annual Data Report: Kidney. *Am. J. Transplant.* **2024**, *24*, S19–S118. [CrossRef] [PubMed]
17. Kasiske, B.L.; Snyder, J.J.; Matas, A.J.; Ellison, M.D.; Gill, J.S.; Kausz, A.T. Preemptive Kidney Transplantation. *J. Am. Soc. Nephrol.* **2002**, *13*, 1358–1364. [CrossRef] [PubMed]
18. Righi, I.; Barone, I.; Rosso, L.; Morlacchi, L.C.; Rossetti, V.; Caffarena, G.; Limanaqi, F.; Palleschi, A.; Clerici, M.; Trabattoni, D. Immunopathology of lung transplantation: From infection to rejection and vice versa. *Front. Immunol.* **2024**, *15*, 1433469. [CrossRef] [PubMed]
19. Austin, P.C.; Stuart, E.A. Moving towards best practice when using inverse probability of treatment weighting (IPTW) using the propensity score to estimate causal treatment effects in observational studies. *Stat. Med.* **2015**, *34*, 3661–3679. [CrossRef] [PubMed]
20. Austin, P.C.; Fine, J.P. Practical recommendations for reporting Fine-Gray model analyses for competing risk data. *Stat. Med.* **2017**, *36*, 4391–4400. [CrossRef] [PubMed]

Journal of
Clinical Medicine

MDPI

Article

Efficacy and Safety of Finerenone in Kidney Transplant Patients

Serdar Kahvecioglu [1,*], Huseyin Celik [2], Asena Serap Yalcinkaya [1], Yavuz Ayar [1], Nimet Aktas [1] and Ozger Akarsu [1]

[1] Nephrology Department, Bursa Yüksek İhtisas Trainig and Research Hospital, Bursa 16310, Turkey; serapp.yalcinkaya@gmail.com (A.S.Y.); yavuzayar@hotmail.com (Y.A.); nimetaktas@gmail.com (N.A.); ozgerakarsu@yahoo.com (O.A.)
[2] Nephrology Department, Bursa Acıbadem Hospital, Bursa 16210, Turkey; huseyin_c66@yahoo.com.tr
* Correspondence: serdarkahvecioglu@hotmail.com

Abstract: Background: Finerenone has emerged as a promising nonsteroidal mineralocorticoid receptor antagonist for patients with chronic kidney disease (CKD), yet its safety and efficacy in kidney transplant recipients remain unstudied. **Methods:** A total of 1750 kidney transplant recipients were screened, and 39 were prescribed finerenone alongside angiotensin-converting enzyme inhibitors or angiotensin II receptor blockers. Fifteen patients who met inclusion criteria and used finerenone consistently for at least six months were compared with 15 matched controls. Proteinuria, renal function, serum potassium, and other laboratory and clinical parameters were assessed at baseline and at 1, 3, and 6 months. **Results:** Finerenone was discontinued in two patients (5.1%) due to flushing and headache. Severe hyperkalemia occurred in four patients (10.2%). In the finerenone group, proteinuria significantly decreased at all time points ($p < 0.05$), with a 40% reduction at six months. No significant changes in estimated glomerular filtration rate or serum creatinine were observed. **Conclusions:** Finerenone is a promising adjunct therapy in kidney transplant patients for reducing proteinuria without impairing renal function for those patients who can tolerate it. However, in the early phase of treatment initiation, patients should be closely monitored for adverse effects including hyperkalemia.

Keywords: finerenone; kidney transplantation; mineralocorticoid receptor antagonists; proteinuria; renal function

1. Introduction

Kidney transplantation is undoubtedly the first treatment option that should be preferred among renal replacement therapies [1]. Although the general condition of patients after kidney transplantation is satisfactory, renal functions may deteriorate due to early and late complications. Many factors such as ischemia reperfusion injury, oxidative stress, toxicity due to drugs used, and recurrence of the primary disease may cause this condition [2]. This deterioration in renal function typically manifests as elevated creatinine levels and proteinuria. Currently, there is no definitive approach to prevent the progression of chronic changes detected by biopsy. In recent years, in patients with chronic kidney disease (CKD) without transplantation, promising results have been achieved with the addition of sodium-glucose co-transporter 2 inhibitors (SGLT2-Is), glucagon-like peptide-1 (GLP-1) agonists, and new-generation nonsteroidal mineralocorticoid receptor antagonists (MRAs) such as finerenone, or combinations of these drugs, in addition with angiotensin-converting enzyme inhibitors (ACEIs) or angiotensin II receptor blockers (ARBs) [3–6]. However, strong evidence on the efficacy and safety of these agents in transplant recipients is required because kidney transplant patients have generally been excluded from major studies. Despite this, favorable results in CKD patients, animal studies, and small-scale clinical trials and case reports suggest that these drugs can also be used in kidney transplant patients [7–11].

Many studies have shown that mineralocorticoid receptors (MRs) become overactive in cardiac and renal diseases [12]. As a result, it has been observed that glomerular and tubular damage in the kidney increases, renal blood flow decreases, and proteinuria increases [13,14]. However, there are also studies showing that vascular and cardiac damage may increase. It has been shown that the use of MRA can be beneficial in blocking this activation [15]. The new generation nonsteroidal MRA finerenone, which binds to MR more effectively and selectively, has no central nervous system penetration and sexual side effects, has very little effect on blood pressure, and has been shown to provide significant benefits in chronic kidney disease [5]. It is thought that its rate of causing hyperkalemia, which is the most feared issue in this group of patients, may be at more acceptable levels compared to other drugs containing MRAs [16,17].

Based on the hypothesis that finerenone could provide beneficial effects such as a reduction in inflammation, fibrosis, oxidative stress, proteinuria, and blood pressure in transplant recipients, we aimed in this study to investigate the efficacy and safety of finerenone in kidney transplant patients.

2. Materials and Methods

2.1. Participants

Our study was conducted by screening a database of 1750 kidney transplant patients from two centers. All patients, regardless of the etiology of the primary kidney disease, both diabetic and non-diabetic, were evaluated.

2.1.1. Inclusion Criteria

Age between 18–65 years.

Having a kidney transplant at least 1 year ago.

Estimated glomerular filtration rate (eGFR) > 25 mL/min.

Receiving ACEI or ARB therapy.

Protein creatinine ratio in spot urine (PCR) > 300 mg/g.

Additionally, patients who had been using 10–20 mg/day active finerenone for at least 6 months and whose baseline serum potassium was not above 5 mg/dL were included in the patient group.

2.1.2. Exclusion Criteria

Rejection episode within the last 3 months.

Surgical intervention within the last 3 months.

Changes in immunosuppressive therapy within the last 3 months.

Receiving albumin infusion.

Unstable clinical condition.

Using potassium-sparing diuretics, potassium supplements, or potassium-lowering treatments.

Active infections.

2.2. Study Design

In this study, which was designed retrospectively, out of the 1750 screened patients, 39 were identified to have been prescribed finerenone at a dose of 10 mg/day.

During follow-up, 15 patients were included in the finerenone group (GROUP 1). Among these, the dose was increased to 20 mg in 10 patients who tolerated the treatment well (according to serum potassium level). An equal number of matched patients meeting inclusion/exclusion criteria and with similar demographic and laboratory parameters were included as the control group (GROUP 2) (Figure 1). A one-to-one matching technique was applied for the pairing of patients and controls according to age, sex, eGFR, and proteinuria levels.

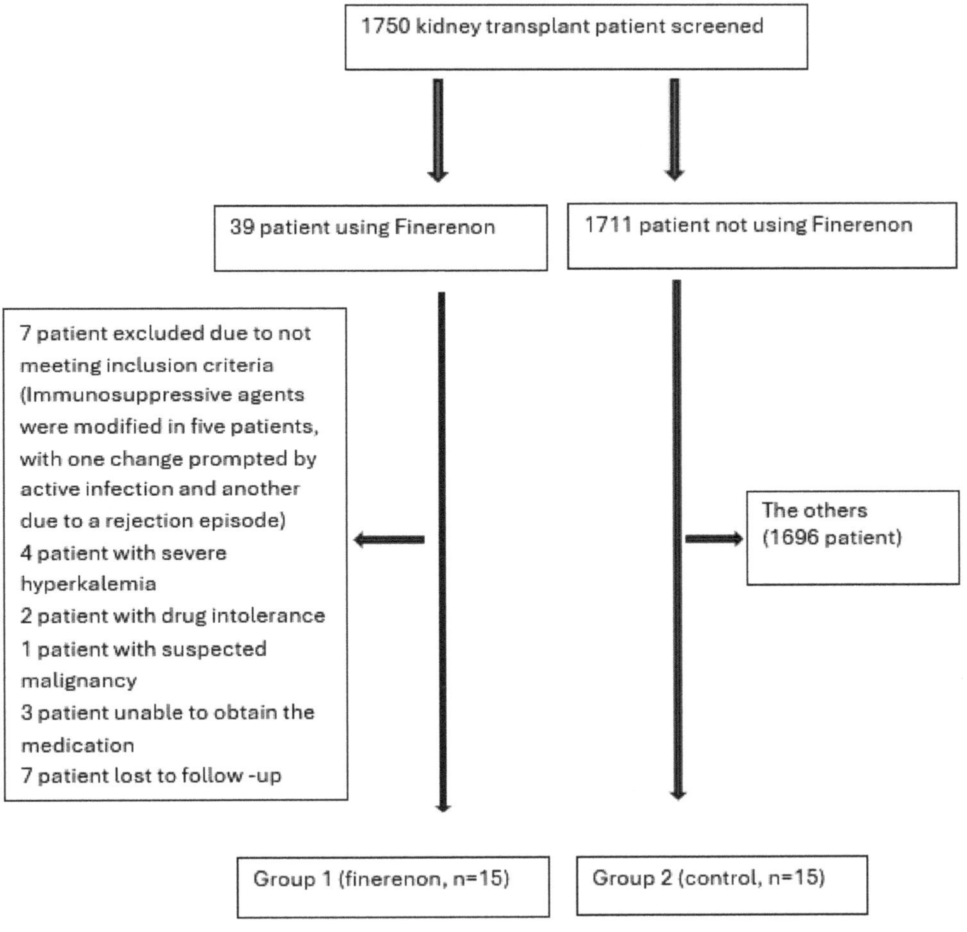

Figure 1. Materials and methods flowchart.

2.3. Data Collection and Follow-Up

The baseline demographic data of the patients in GROUP 1 who used finerenone and were included in the study, such as kidney transplantation type, presence of diabetes, serum urea, serum creatinine, serum potassium, eGFR, uric acid, alanine amino transferase, and the medications they used, were recorded from the routine visit information on the day treatment with finerenone was started. The data from the visits of the patients who used their medication regularly, which were closest to the 1st, 3rd, and 6th months, were also taken for evaluation. The patients in GROUP 2, who were included as the control group, were selected if their clinical conditions were stable and their proteinuria, eGFR, potassium levels, and demographic characteristics were compatible. The first value of these patients was accepted as the starting point in order to fit the averages of the patient group.

The laboratory and demographic data from the closest follow-up visits at the 1st, 3rd, and 6th months were recorded. eGFR values were calculated according to the Chronic Kidney Disease Epidemiology Collaboration (CKD-EPI) formula, and proteinuria was calculated according to the protein/creatinine ratio in spot urine. Blood pressure assessment was not performed due to the lack of standardization, including differences in measurement devices, variability among personnel conducting the measurements, and incomplete documentation in patient records.

2.4. Ethics Statement

The study was approved by a local ethics committee on 26.03.2025 (decision number 2024-TBEK 2025/03-05). The study adhered to the Declaration of Helsinki and Good Clinical Practice guidelines.

2.5. Data Analysis

Data were collected from electronic medical records. Normality of continuous variables was tested using the Shapiro–Wilk test. Descriptive statistics were presented as percentages for categorical variables and as median, minimum–maximum, and 25th–75th percentiles for continuous variables.

For repeated measures within dependent groups, the Friedman test was used. If the Friedman test indicated statistical significance, post hoc pairwise comparisons were performed using the Wilcoxon signed-rank test. Categorical variables between groups were compared using the Chi-square test. Bonferroni correction was applied for multiple comparisons.

All statistical analyses were performed using IBM SPSS Statistics version 26.0 (IBM Corp., Armonk, NY, USA). A type I error rate of 5% ($p < 0.05$) was considered statistically significant.

3. Results

In the study, data were obtained from 15 patients who met the inclusion and exclusion criteria and used finerenone and 15 control patients with compatible demographic and laboratory data from 1750 kidney transplant patients (Figure 1). In the finerenone group, the median age was 42 (24–61) years, the transplantation period was 58 (13–150) months, and 33% of the patients were female, while in the control group, the mean age was 45 (19–59) years, the transplantation period was 80 (12–142) months, and 60% of the patients were female ($p > 0.05$). In the finerenone group, 1 patient and in the control group, 2 patients were using cyclosporine + mycophenolate mofetil + low-dose steroids, and all other patients were using tacrolimus + mycophenolate mofetil + low-dose steroids. There was no statistically significant difference in baseline values between the groups ($p > 0.05$) (Table 1).

A statistically significant decrease in proteinuria was found in the patients using finerenone; this was more pronounced in the 1st month ($p < 0.002$) throughout the follow-up period ($p < 0.05$). This decrease in proteinuria in the finerenone group was at the level of 40% at the end of the 6-month follow-up. There was no significant difference compared to the control group (Figure 2, Table 2).

Table 1. Descriptive statics of clinical and biochemical parameters by groups.

Variables	Finerenon (n = 15) Median (Min–Max)	Control (n = 15) Median (Min–Max)	p
Age (years)	42 (24–61)	45 (19–59)	>0.05
Weight (kg)	75 (50–110)	70 (44.60–111)	>0.05
Height (cm)	170 (153–190)	171 (158–190)	>0.05
Transplant duration (months)	58 (13–150)	80 (12–142)	>0.05
BUN (mg/dL)	24 (14–49)	23(13–42)	>0.05
Creatinine (mg/dL)	1.85 (1.00–3.34)	1.52 (1.12–2.38)	>0.05
eGFR (mL/min/1.73 m^2)	41.7 (25.80–81.17)	48.31(26.80–84.66)	>0.05
Proteinuria (mg/day)	2150 (600–5335)	1691 (403–7112)	>0.05
Uric acid (mg/dL)	6.9 (4.75–12.11)	6.7 (4.82–11.40)	>0.05
Potassium (mmol/L)	4.35 (3.29–5.00)	4.22 (3.30–5.00)	>0.05
ALT (U/L)	14 (5–36)	17 (8–33)	>0.05
LDL (mg/dL)	103 (38–257)	103 (40–215)	>0.05
TG (mg/dL)	147 (80–787)	101 (68–451)	>0.05
Tacrolimus (ng/mL)	7.70 (4.30–10.25)	6.52 (3.14–9.9)	>0.05
Donor Type (Living/Deceased)	11/4	7/8	>0.05
Sex (F/M)	5/10	9/6	>0.05
Smoking (+/−)	5/10	3/12	>0.05
Etiology			
HTN	9	12	
DM	1	0	
DM + HTN	1	0	
Others	4	1	
Unknown	0	2	

Notes: min: minimum value, max: maximum value. Abbreviations: eGFR: estimated glomerular filtration rate, F: female, M: male, ALT: alanine aminotransferase, BUN: blood urea nitrogen, HTN: hypertension, DM: diabetes mellitus, GN: glomerulonephritis, LDL: low-density lipoprotein, TG: triglyceride.

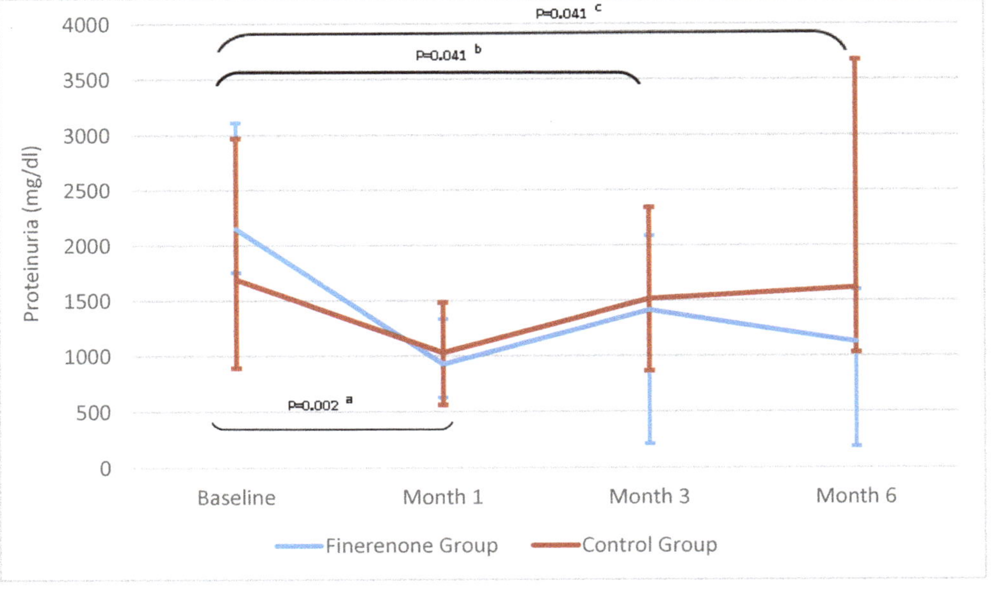

Figure 2. Changes in proteinuria over time. Data are presented as median (25p–75p). [a] Baseline–month 1 in GROUP 1, [b] Baseline–month 3 in GROUP 1, [c] Baseline–month 6 in GROUP 1.

Table 2. Statistical distribution of baseline and 6th-month data in the finerenon and control groups.

Variables	GROUP 1 Median (Min–Max) Baseline	6th Month	p *	GROUP 2 Median (Min–Max) Baseline	6th Month	p &	p #
BUN (mg/dL)	24 (14–49)	26 (17–53)	>0.05	23 (13–42)	26 (18–72)	>0.05	>0.05
Creatinine (mg/dL)	1.85 (1–3.34)	1.82 (1–3.95)	>0.05	1.52 (1.12–2.38)	1.68 (0.91–4.26)	**<0.05**	>0.05
eGFR (mL/dk/1.73 m^2)	41.7 (25.8–81.1)	40 (19.2–83.5)	>0.05	48.3 (26.80–84.66)	48.7 (17.00–69.35)	**<0.05**	>0.05
Proteinuria (mg/day)	2150 (600–5335)	1127 (80–3848)	**<0.05**	1691(403–7112)	1615 (420–5389)	>0.05	>0.05
Potassium (mmol/L)	4.35 (3.29–5)	4.32 (3.4–4.7)	>0.05	4.20 (3.3–5.0)	4.4 (3.4–5.5)	>0.05	>0.05
Tacrolimus (ng/mL)	7.7 (4.3–10.25)	6.28 (3.66–10.5)	>0.05	6.52 (3.14–9.9)	6.2 (4.7–10.2)	>0.05	>0.05
Uric acid (mg/dL)	6.9 (4.15–12.1)	6.27 (4.4–10.54)	>0.05	6.27 (4.82–11.4)	6 (4.96–10.8)	>0.05	>0.05
ALT (IU/L)	14 (5–36)	17 (5–58)	>0.05	13 (8–33)	16 (5–69)	>0.05	>0.05
LDL (mg/dL)	103 (38–257)	112 (36–191)	>0.05	103 (40–215)	115 (36–207)	>0.05	>0.05
TG (mg/dL)	147 (80–787)	173 (50–466)	>0.05	101 (70–502)	159 (37–581)	>0.05	>0.05

Notes: *: between baseline and 6th month in GROUP 1, &: between baseline and 6th month in GROUP 2, #: between groups, min: minimum value, max: maximum value. Abbreviations: BUN: blood urea nitrogen, eGFR: estimated glomerular filtration rate, ALT: alanine aminotransferase, LDL: low-density lipoprotein, TG: triglyceride.

The Friedman test showed a significant difference among the three time points in GROUP 1 ($\chi^2 = 13.588$, $p = 0.004$). Post hoc Wilcoxon signed-rank tests revealed significant differences between baseline and the first month ($p = 0.002$), between baseline and the third month ($p = 0.041$), and between baseline and the sixth month ($p = 0.041$), but not between the third and sixth months ($p = 0.43$), after Bonferroni correction.

In terms of renal functions, it was observed that creatinine levels increased slightly in the first month in the finerenone group ($p = 0.055$) but decreased to near-baseline levels in the 3rd and 6th months. The change in eGFR was not statistically significant and remained stable. In the control group, there was a significant creatinine increase compared to the baseline in the 1st and 6th months. Statistical significance was found in eGFR compared to the baseline in the 6th month ($p = 0.023$). No significant difference was found in the comparison between the groups ($p > 0.05$) (Figures 3 and 4, Table 2).

When all patients who were started on finerenone were considered, the drug was discontinued due to side effects (flashing and headache) in 2 out of 39 patients (5.1%). One of the most curious issues when using MRA, significant hyperkalemia (>6 mEq/L) occurred in 4 (10.2) patients, and the drug was discontinued. During the treatment, it was observed that 3 out of 15 patients in the finerenone group with a baseline value of ≤5 mEq/L had asymptomatic mild potassium elevation in the 1st month (maximum 5.7 mEq/L), and 3 patients in the 3rd month (maximum 5.5 mEq/L). The potassium increase in the 1st month was significant, and there was a decrease toward the initial levels in the 3rd and 6th months (≤5 mEq/L). There were no patients with hyperkalemia leading to death, hospitalization, or dialysis. When the potassium changes in the 1st, 3rd, and 6th months of the study were compared with the control group, it was observed that there was no statistical difference ($p > 0.05$) (Figure 5, Table 2).

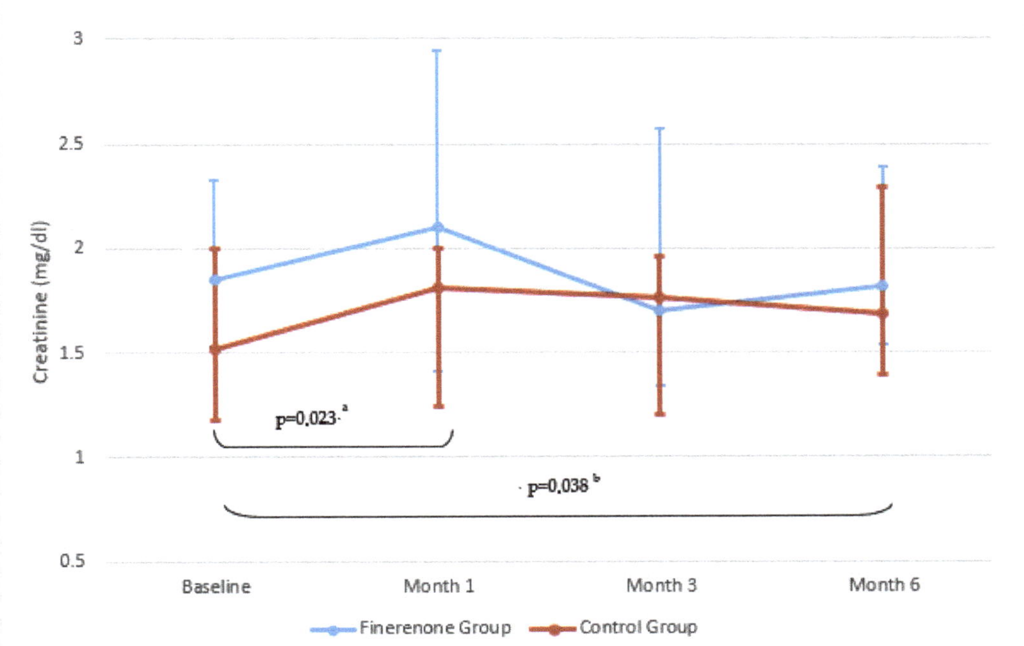

Figure 3. Changes in serum creatinine over time. Data are presented as median (25p–75p). [a] Baseline–month 1 in GROUP 2, [b] Baseline–month 6 in GROUP 2, creatinine levels showed a statistically significant decrease from baseline to 1 month (Z = −2.273, p = 0.023) and from baseline to 6 months (Z = −2.074, p = 0.038).

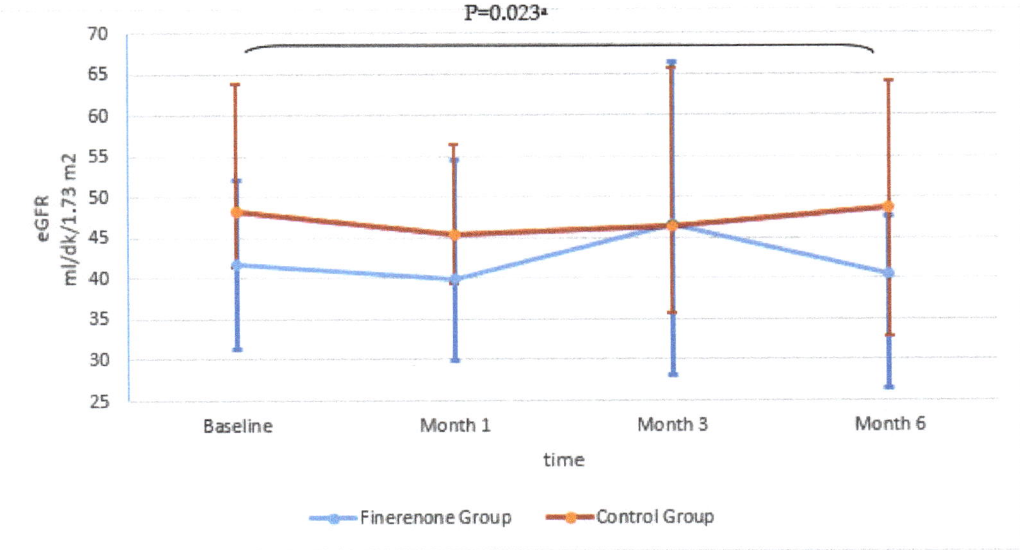

Figure 4. Changes in serum estimated glomerular filtration rate (eGFR) over time. Data are presented as median (25p–75p). [a] Baseline–month 6 in GROUP 2, eGFR levels showed a statistically significant decrease from baseline to 6 months (Z = −2.272, p = 0.023).

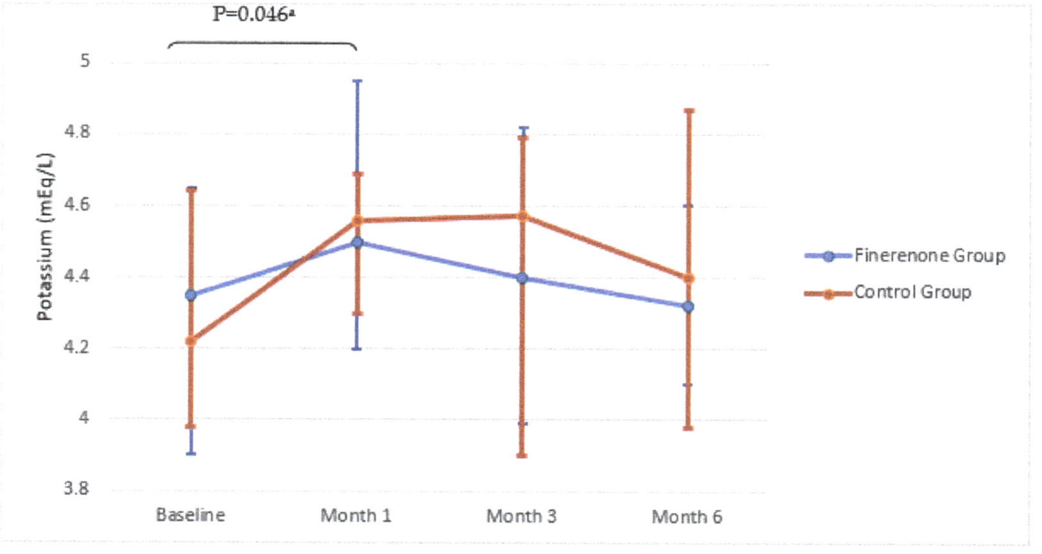

Figure 5. Changes in serum potassium over time. Data are presented as median (25p–75p). [a] Baseline–month 1 in GROUP 1. In GROUP 1, potassium levels showed a statistically significant increase from baseline to 1 month ($Z = -1.992$, $p = 0.046$).

We did not find any statistical difference in the use of finerenone in patients using tacrolimus in terms of drug level in the comparison between groups or within the groups ($p > 0.05$). The comparisons of other laboratory parameters are shown in Table 2.

4. Discussion

This study is the first to investigate the potential efficacy of finerenone in kidney transplant recipients.

The presence of proteinuria is one of the main indicators of kidney damage in kidney transplant recipients, as in kidney diseases [18,19]. Studies have shown that proteinuria can be observed in up to 40% of kidney transplant recipients [20]. Many guidelines state that the use of SGLT2I, GLP1 agonist, or finerenone, or their combination therapies in addition to ARBs, especially in chronic kidney disease patients with heart failure or diabetes, are beneficial and should be added to treatment algorithms [4,21,22]. However, since kidney transplant patients were considered as an exclusion criterion in all large studies conducted with drugs known to be effective in renal protection, we did not have studies to guide us [5]. In our evaluation of the 15 patients who used finerenone and had regular follow-ups among the 1750 kidney transplant patients that we followed, and the same number of control group patients who did not have any statistical differences between them, we found that the use of finerenone provided a 40% decrease in proteinuria at the end of the 6-month follow-up and that this decrease was statistically significant compared to the baseline throughout the follow-up period, especially in the first month. In a meta-analysis evaluating 19 studies, it was observed that finerenone added to renin-angiotensin-aldosterone system blockers in non-transplant chronic kidney disease patients provided a 38.7% decrease in proteinuria, and the fact that almost the same result was obtained in our study suggests that the drug may be effective in kidney transplant patients as in non-transplant CKD [8,23]. As in the FIGARO-DKD study, it is observed that the effectiveness of the drug increases as the amount of proteinuria increases [5,23,24]. In a retrospective study conducted with spironolactone, a nonselective MRA, in kidney transplant recipients, it was detected that a statistically significant decrease in proteinuria was achieved after 6 months of treatment in patients with proteinuria over 1 g [8]. The fact that the average proteinuria was over 2 g/day in our study supports these studies and may have contributed to our results being more significant.

When we look at eGFR, which is one of the main indicators in the evaluation of renal functions, a slight decrease in eGFR was observed in the finerenone group as of the first month after starting the drug, and it returned to baseline values by the end of the sixth month. Serum creatinine also has a course parallel to eGFR, and the significant creatinine increase detected in the control group at the end of the six-month follow-up was not seen in the group receiving the drug. This situation observed in our kidney transplant patients is similar to the findings in studies conducted in other CKD groups without kidney transplantation. There are studies showing that MRAs are effective, especially in patients with eGFR values >30 mL/min/1.73 m^2, and that this effect decreases as eGFR decreases [25–28]. When the data of the FIDELITY study, conducted with finerenone and examining over 13,000 CKD stage 1–4 patients, were evaluated, it was determined that there was a significant benefit in renal outcomes, including GFR, in the group receiving the drug [8]. In the recently concluded SPIREN study, which investigated renal function, proteinuria, and renal allotransplant fibrosis with the addition of spironolactone, a nonselective MRA, to standard treatment in kidney transplant recipients, with a follow-up of 3 years, no significant benefit was found [29]. However, there is no study conducted with selective MRAs. In our study, it was observed that the use of finerenone in kidney transplant patients, as in other chronic kidney disease patients, did not have at least a negative effect on eGFR, and the significant creatinine increase seen in the control group was not observed in the group receiving the drug.

The most feared condition in all studies conducted with MRAs is hyperkalemia. ACEIs and ARBs are generally used intensively in patients with impaired renal function or proteinuria. This situation further increases the risk of hyperkalemia. It has been shown that MRAs have a greater risk of hyperkalemia, especially in patients with high proteinuria, low GFR, and high baseline potassium levels [30,31]. Several studies have shown that finerenone causes significantly less hyperkalemia compared with spironolactone [32,33]. The main reasons for this may be the short half-life of the drug, the absence of active metabolites, and the mechanism of action of MR, which includes different receptor blockades and gene expression in organs such as the kidney and heart [34]. Finerenone is also superior to spironolactone in terms of gynecomastia [29,35]. In our study, severe hyperkalemia occurred in 10.4% of patients starting finerenone. Compared to the FIDELITY (1.7%) and FINE-REAL (5%) studies, our study demonstrated a higher risk of hyperkalemia [24,36]. However, mild asymptomatic hyperkalemia at early follow-up resolved over time, and overall potassium changes were not significantly different from controls. Given the high incidence of hyperkalemia, it was concluded that finerenone should be initiated at the lowest possible dose in transplant patients, with closer monitoring required compared to other patient populations.

There is no comprehensive study examining the effects of finerenone use on the serum levels of calcineurin inhibitors in organ transplant patients. Calcineurin inhibitors are drugs that significantly provide graft survival in organ transplant patients. However, they may have toxic effects at plasma levels outside the therapeutic range. At the same time, these drugs may cause calcineurin inhibitor-associated nephrotoxicity due to reducing renal blood flow, increasing oxidative stress, upregulating transforming growth factor-beta, and activating apoptotic genes [37–39]. It is thought that finerenone may have a positive effect on these pathological mechanisms. In an animal study on this subject, it was shown that finerenone added to standard treatment provided significant benefits in creatinine, interleukin-6, urinary neutrophil gelatinase-associated lipocalin, and blood pressure levels in a tacrolimus-mediated renal failure model compared to the group not receiving the drug [40]. In our study, no statistically significant difference was detected in the tacrolimus level at the 6-month follow-up. Long-term studies including histopathological evaluation are needed to examine the effects of finerenone on calcineurin-mediated nephropathy.

There are many etiological factors that can impair renal functions in organ transplant patients. The main ones are ischemia reperfusion injury, delayed graft function, rejection attacks, and calcineurin toxicity. It is known that MR is upregulated in many cases where renal damage occurs [12]. Based on this point, we think that the renoprotection shown in patients with CKD, whether diabetic or not, with the use of finerenone may also benefit organ transplant patients. However, considering the medications used in transplant recipients and patient-specific factors, aspects such as the pharmacokinetics of finerenone, its interactions with immunosuppressive agents, and the presence of various underlying causes of proteinuria require further elucidation. Although there is no published study on this subject, the ongoing EFFEKTOR (NCT06059664) study is an important study that will show the efficacy and safety of finerenone in kidney transplant recipients. Again, two studies (NCT02490904, NCT04450953) are ongoing to evaluate eplerenone in kidney transplant patients.

The most important limitation of our study is its retrospective design, which did not include randomization of subjects between the finerenone and control groups. Thus, there may have been differences between these groups accounting for the differences in proteinuria unrelated to taking finerenone. Additional limitations include the small number of cases, short follow-up period, retrospective data collection, lack of blood pressure monitoring, adjustment for confounding variables, and lack of biopsy data.

In conclusion, this study suggests that finerenone may contribute to the reduction of proteinuria in renal transplant patients as part of their therapeutic management and had no negative effect on GFR. Our study also identified a 15% dropout rate due to adverse events: 5% due to headache and flushing and 10% due to a risk of hyperkalemia, especially during the early phases of drug initiation, underscoring the importance of dose potassium surveillance. Prospective, randomized, controlled studies with large case series are needed on this subject.

Author Contributions: S.K., H.C. and A.S.Y. were responsible for study planning and execution. Y.A. contributed to the manuscript as the English language editor. N.A. and O.A. assisted in the collection and evaluation of the data. All authors have read and agreed to the published version of the manuscript.

Funding: This research received no external funding.

Institutional Review Board Statement: The study was approved by the Ethics Committee of Bursa Yüksek İhtisas Training and Research Hospital on 26 March 2025 (decision number 2024-TBEK 2025/03-05). The study adhered to the Declaration of Helsinki and Good Clinical Practice guidelines.

Informed Consent Statement: Informed consent was obtained from all subjects involved in the study.

Data Availability Statement: The data that support the findings of this study are available from the corresponding author upon reasonable request.

Acknowledgments: We gratefully acknowledge the contributions of all clinical staff and research coordinators involved in patient recruitment and data collection. We extend our sincere appreciation to the nephrology department for their unwavering support throughout this study. Special thanks to our patients, whose participation made this research possible. We thanks to Pinar Ozdemir for her statical studies.

Conflicts of Interest: The authors declare no conflicts of interest.

Abbreviations

ACEIs	Angiotensin-converting Enzyme Inhibitors
ARBs	Angiotensin II Receptor Blockers
CKD	Chronic Kidney Disease
CKD-EPI	The Chronic Kidney Disease Epidemiology Collaboration
eGFR	Estimated Glomerular Filtration Rate
GFR	Glomerüler Filtration Rate
GLP-1	Glucagon-like Peptide-1
MRAs	Nonsteroidal Mineralocorticoid Receptor Antagonists
MR	Mineralocorticoid Receptor
SGLT2-Is	Sodium-glucose Co-transporter 2 Inhibitors

References

1. Chaudhry, D.; Chaudhry, A.; Peracha, J.; Sharif, A. Survival for waitlisted kidney failure patients receiving transplantation versus remaining on waiting list: Systematic review and meta-analysis. *BMJ* **2002**, *376*, e068769. [CrossRef]
2. Minkovich, M.; Gupta, N.; Liu, M.; Famure, O.; Li, Y.; Selzner, M.; Lee, J.Y.; Kim, S.J.; Ghanekar, A. Impact of early surgical complications on kidney transplant outcomes. *BMC Surg.* **2024**, *24*, 165. [CrossRef]
3. American Diabetes Association Professional Practice Committee. 11. Chronic kidney disease and risk management: Standards of care in diabetes–2024. *Diabetes Care* **2024**, *47*, S219–S230. [CrossRef]
4. de Boer, I.H.; Khunti, K.; Sadusky, T.; Tuttle, K.R.; Neumiller, J.J.; Rhee, C.M.; Rosas, S.E.; Rossing, P.; Bakris, G. Diabetes management in chronic kidney disease: A consensus report by the American Diabetes Association (ADA) and Kidney Disease: Improving Global Outcomes (KDIGO). *Diabetes Care* **2022**, *45*, 3075–3090. [CrossRef] [PubMed]
5. Pitt, B.; Filippatos, G.; Agarwal, R.; Anker, S.D.; Bakris, G.L.; Rossing, P.; Joseph, A.; Kolkhof, P.; Nowack, C.; Schloemer, P.; et al. Cardiovascular events with finerenone in kidney disease and type 2 diabetes. *N. Engl. J. Med.* **2021**, *385*, 2252–2263. [CrossRef] [PubMed]
6. Bakris, G.L.; Agarwal, R.; Anker, S.D.; Pitt, B.; Ruilope, L.M.; Rossing, P.; Kolkhof, P.; Nowack, C.; Schloemer, P.; Joseph, A.; et al. Effect of finerenone on chronic kidney disease outcomes in type 2 diabetes. *N. Engl. J. Med.* **2020**, *383*, 2219–2229. [CrossRef]
7. Abdelhakim, A.M.; Abd-ElGawad, M. Impact of mineralocorticoid receptor antagonist in renal transplant patients: A systematic review and meta-analysis of randomized controlled trials. *J. Nephrol.* **2020**, *33*, 529–538. [CrossRef]
8. de Sousa, M.; Guida, J.; Valle, C.D.; Camargo, L.; Rivelli, G.; Mazzali, M. Spironolactone in post-transplant proteinuria: A safe alternative therapy. *Transplant. Proc.* **2017**, *49*, 813–816. [CrossRef] [PubMed]
9. Baskin, E.; Alam Siddiqui, M.; Gülleroğlu, K.; Özdemir, B.H.; Yılmaz, A.Ç.; Çolak, M.Y.; Akdur, A.; Soy, E.A.; Moray, G.; Haberal, M. Long-term effect of eplerenone treatment in children with chronic allograft nephropathy. *Pediatr. Transplant.* **2023**, *27*, e14557. [CrossRef]
10. Waanders, F.; Rienstra, H.; Boer, M.W.; Zandvoort, A.; Rozing, J.; Navis, G.; van Goor, H.; Hillebrands, J.-L. Spironolactone ameliorates transplant vasculopathy in renal chronic transplant dysfunction in rats. *Am. J. Physiol. Renal Physiol.* **2009**, *296*, F1072–F1079. [CrossRef]
11. Afsar, B.; Afsar, R.E.; Caliskan, Y.; Lentine, K.L. Mineralocorticoid receptor blockage in kidney transplantation: Too much of a good thing or not? *Int. Urol. Nephrol.* **2025**, *57*, 839–854. [CrossRef]
12. Buonafine, M.; Bonnard, B.; Jaisser, F. Roles of mineralocorticoid receptors in cardiovascular and cardiorenal diseases. *Am. J. Hypertens.* **2018**, *31*, 1165–1174. [CrossRef] [PubMed]
13. Kolkhof, P.; Lawatscheck, R.; Filippatos, G.; Bakris, G.L. Nonsteroidal mineralocorticoid receptor antagonism by finerenone-translational aspects and clinical perspectives across multiple organ systems. *Int. J. Mol. Sci.* **2022**, *23*, 9243. [CrossRef] [PubMed]
14. Kolkhof, P.; Joseph, A.; Kintscher, U. Nonsteroidal mineralocorticoid receptor antagonism for cardiovascular and renal disorders—New perspectives for combination therapy. *Pharmacol. Res.* **2021**, *172*, 105859. [CrossRef]
15. Barrera-Chimal, J.; Lima-Posada, I.; Bakris, G.L.; Jaisser, F. Mineralocorticoid receptor antagonists in diabetic kidney disease—Mechanistic and therapeutic effects. *Nat. Rev. Nephrol.* **2022**, *18*, 56–70. [CrossRef]
16. Bakris, G.; E Pergola, P.; Delgado, B.; Genov, D.; Doliashvili, T.; Vo, N.; Yang, Y.F.; McCabe, J.; Benn, V.; Pitt, B. Effect of KBP-5074 on blood pressure in advanced chronic kidney disease: Results of the BLOCK-CKD study. *Hypertension* **2021**, *78*, 74–81. [CrossRef] [PubMed]

17. Jaisser, F.; Barrera-Chimal, J. Mineralocorticoid receptor antagonism for non-diabetic kidney disease. *Nephrol. Dial. Transplant.* **2025**, *40*, i29–i36. [CrossRef]
18. Hemmelgarn, B.R.; Manns, B.J.; Lloyd, A.; James, M.T.; Klarenbach, S.; Quinn, R.R.; Wiebe, N.; Tonelli, M.; Alberta Kidney Disease Network. Relation between kidney function, proteinuria, and adverse outcomes. *JAMA* **2010**, *303*, 423–429. [CrossRef]
19. Fernández-Fresnedo, G.; Escallada, R.; Rodrigo, E.; De Francisco, A.L.; Cotorruelo, J.G.; De Castro, S.S.; Zubimendi, J.A.; Ruiz, J.C.; Arias, M. The risk of cardiovascular disease associated with proteinuria in renal transplant patients. *Transplantation* **2002**, *73*, 1345–1348. [CrossRef]
20. Shamseddin, M.K.; Knoll, G.A. Posttransplantation proteinuria: An approach to diagnosis and management. *Clin. J. Am. Soc. Nephrol.* **2011**, *6*, 1786–1793. [CrossRef]
21. Kidney Disease: Improving Global Outcomes (KDIGO) CKD Work Group. KDIGO 2024 clinical practice guideline for the evaluation and management of chronic kidney disease. *Kidney Int.* **2024**, *105* (Suppl. 4), S117–S314. [CrossRef]
22. Agarwal, R.; Green, J.B.; Heerspink, H.J.; Mann, J.F.; McGill, J.B.; Mottl, A.K.; Rosenstock, J.; Rossing, P.; Vaduganathan, M.; Brinker, M.; et al. Finerenone with Empagliflozin in Chronic Kidney Disease and Type 2 Diabetes. *N. Engl. J. Med.* **2025**, *393*, 533–543. [CrossRef]
23. Currie, G.; Taylor, A.H.M.; Fujita, T.; Ohtsu, H.; Lindhardt, M.; Rossing, P.; Boesby, L.; Edwards, N.C.; Ferro, C.J.; Townend, J.N.; et al. Effect of mineralocorticoid receptor antagonists on proteinuria and progression of chronic kidney disease: A systematic review and meta-analysis. *BMC Nephrol.* **2016**, *17*, 127. [CrossRef]
24. Nicholas, S.B.; Correa-Rotter, R.; Desai, N.R.; Guo, L.; Navaneethan, S.D.; Pantalone, K.M.; Wanner, C.; Hamacher, S.; Fatoba, S.T.; Horvat-Broecker, A.; et al. First interim results from FINE-REAL: A prospective, non-interventional, phase 4 study providing insights into the use and safety of finerenone in a routine clinical setting. *J. Nephrol.* **2024**, *7*, 2223–2232. [CrossRef] [PubMed]
25. Ferreira, J.P.; Pitt, B.; McMurray, J.J.; Pocock, S.J.; Solomon, S.D.; Pfeffer, M.A.; Zannad, F.; Rossignol, P. Steroidal MRA Across the Spectrum of Renal Function: A Pooled Analysis of RCTs. *JACC Heart Fail.* **2022**, *10*, 842–850. [CrossRef] [PubMed]
26. Oh, J.; Kang, S.-M.; Song, M.K.; Hong, N.; Youn, J.-C.; Han, S.; Jeon, E.-S.; Cho, M.-C.; Kim, J.-J.; Yoo, B.-S.; et al. Clinical Benefit of Spironolactone in Patients with Acute Decompensated Heart Failure and Severe Renal Dysfunction: Data from the Korean Heart Failure Registry. *Am. Heart J.* **2015**, *169*, 713–720.e3. [CrossRef] [PubMed]
27. Tseng, W.-C.; Liu, J.-S.; Hung, S.-C.; Kuo, K.-L.; Chen, Y.-H.; Tarng, D.-C.; Hsu, C.-C. Effect of Spironolactone on the Risks of Mortality and Hospitalization for Heart Failure in Pre-Dialysis Advanced Chronic kidney Disease: A Nationwide Population-Based Study. *Int. J. Cardiol.* **2017**, *238*, 72–78. [CrossRef]
28. Inampudi, C.; Parvataneni, S.; Morgan, C.J.; Deedwania, P.; Fonarow, G.C.; Sanders, P.W.; Prabhu, S.D.; Butler, J.; Forman, D.E.; Aronow, W.S.; et al. Spironolactone Use and Higher Hospital Readmission for Medicare Beneficiaries with Heart Failure, LeftVentricular Ejection Fraction <45%, and Estimated Glomerular Filtration Rate <45 ml/min/1.73 m2. Am. *J. Cardiol.* **2014**, *114*, 79–82.
29. Mortensen, L.A.; Jespersen, B.; Helligsoe, A.S.L.; Tougaard, B.; Cibulskyte-Ninkovic, D.; Egfjord, M.; Boesby, L.; Marcussen, N.; Madsen, K.; Jensen, B.L.; et al. Effect of Spironolactone on Kidney Function in Kidney Transplant Recipients (the SPIREN trial): A Randomized Placebo-Controlled Clinical Trial. *Clin. J. Am. Soc. Nephrol.* **2024**, *19*, 755–766. [CrossRef]
30. Kovesdy, C.P.; Matsushita, K.; Sang, Y.; Brunskill, N.J.; Carrero, J.J.; Chodick, G.; Hasegawa, T.; Heerspink, H.L.; Hirayama, A.; Landman, G.W.D.; et al. Serum potassium and adverse outcomes across the range of kidney function: A CKD prognosis consortium meta-analysis. *Eur. Heart J.* **2018**, *39*, 1535–1542. [CrossRef]
31. Clase, C.M.; Carrero, J.-J.; Ellison, D.H.; Grams, M.E.; Hemmelgarn, B.R.; Jardine, M.J.; Kovesdy, C.P.; Kline, G.A.; Lindner, G.; Obrador, G.T.; et al. Potassium homeostasis and management of dyskalemia in kidney diseases: Conclusions from a Kidney Disease: Improving Global Outcomes (KDIGO) Controversies Conference. Available online: https://kdigo.org/wp-content/uploads/2018/04/KDIGO-Potassium-Management-Final-publication.pdf. (accessed on 9 December 2021).
32. Epstein, M.; Williams, G.H.; Weinberger, M.; Lewin, A.; Krause, S.; Mukherjee, R.; Patni, R.; Beckerman, B. Selective aldosterone blockade with eplerenone reduces albuminuria in patients with type 2 diabetes. *Clin. J. Am. Soc. Nephrol.* **2006**, *1*, 940–951. [CrossRef] [PubMed]
33. Pitt, B.; Kober, L.; Ponikowski, P.; Gheorghiade, M.; Filippatos, G.; Krum, H.; Nowack, C.; Kolkhof, P.; Kim, S.-Y.; Zannad, F. Safety and tolerability of the novel non-steroidal mineralocorticoid receptor antagonist BAY 94-8862 in patients with chronic heart failure and mild or moderate chronic kidney disease: A randomized, double-blind trial. *Eur. Heart J.* **2013**, *34*, 2453–2463. [CrossRef]
34. Agarwal, R.; Kolkhof, P.; Bakris, G.; Bauersachs, J.; Haller, H.; Wada, T.; Zannad, F. Steroidal and non-steroidal mineralocorticoid receptor antagonists in cardiorenal medicine. *Eur. Heart J.* **2021**, *42*, 152–161. [CrossRef]
35. Pitt, B.; Pfeffer, M.A.; Assmann, S.F.; Boineau, R.; Anand, I.S.; Claggett, B.; Clausell, N.; Desai, A.S.; Diaz, R.; Fleg, J.L.; et al. Spironolactone for heart failure with preserved ejection fraction. *N. Engl. J. Med.* **2014**, *370*, 1383–1392. [CrossRef]
36. Desai, N.R.; Navaneethan, S.D.; Nicholas, S.B.; Pantalone, K.M.; Wanner, C.; Hamacher, S.; Gay, A.; Wheeler, D.C. Design and rationale of FINE-REAL: A prospective study of finerenone in clinical practice. *J. Diabetes Complicat.* **2023**, *37*, 108411. [CrossRef]

37. Nankivell, B.J.; P'Ng, C.H.; O'Connell, P.J.; Chapman, J.R. Calcineurin inhibitor nephrotoxicity through the lens of longitudinal histology: Comparison of cyclosporine and tacrolimus eras. *Transplantation* **2016**, *100*, 1723–1731. [CrossRef]
38. Feria, I.; Pichardo, I.; Juárez, P.; Ramírez, V.; González, M.A.; Uribe, N.; García-Torres, R.; López-Casillas, F.; Gamba, G.; Bobadilla, N.A. Therapeutic benefit of spironolactone in experimental chronic cyclosporine a nephrotoxicity. *Kidney Int.* **2003**, *63*, 43–52. [CrossRef] [PubMed]
39. Kanbay, M.; Copur, S.; Mizrak, B.; Mallamaci, F.; Zoccali, C. Mineralocorticoid receptor antagonists in kidney transplantation. *Eur. J. Clin. Investig.* **2024**, *54*, e14206. [CrossRef] [PubMed]
40. Figueroa, S.M.; Bertocchio, J.-P.; Nakamura, T.; El-Moghrabi, S.; Jaisser, F.; Amador, C.A. The Mineralocorticoid Receptor on Smooth Muscle Cells Promotes Tacrolimus-Induced Renal Injury in Mice. *Pharmaceutics* **2023**, *15*, 1373. [CrossRef] [PubMed]

MDPI AG
Grosspeteranlage 5
4052 Basel
Switzerland
Tel.: +41 61 683 77 34

Journal of Clinical Medicine Editorial Office
E-mail: jcm@mdpi.com
www.mdpi.com/journal/jcm

www.ingramcontent.com/pod-product-compliance
Lightning Source LLC
Chambersburg PA
CBHW062058220926
51850CB00010B/2814
9783725869664